ENDORSEMENTS
FOR : PLAY YOUR HAND WELL

"This excellent book on how we can control much of our health destiny is the first from Dr. Mix. I hope there will be more to come. Special touches noted in the book include supplements that may be especially useful for oral hygiene. Also, the inside look at conducting a clinical trial with ginkgo will be of interest to many. I would recommend this book to all who are interested in enhancing their health."

Jerry M. Cott, Ph.D., Psychopharmacology, Fulton, Maryland

Former Chief of Psychopharmacology Research Program, NIMH

"Finally, a nutrition book that is both very informative, yet easy to read and apply. As an exercise physiologist, I am often asked questions regarding nutrition. I feel that I can wholeheartedly recommend this book to my clients and know that they will be getting quality information. Best of all, the Mix Food Index actually gives us a way to compare apples and oranges."

Dr. Jim Schoffstall, RCEP

Registered Clinical Exercise Physiologist

"Informational, applicable, entertaining, and inspiring best describe the material Dr. Mix has assembled in his book. There are many nutrition books on the market; however, what sets this book apart from others is the manner in which the author has taken concepts that often seem confusing and complicated and presents them in a way that is not only easy to understand, but also applicable to everyday life. This book will help anyone to begin and continue a lifespan of healthy living through knowledge and appreciation of nutrition and exercise."

Mike Sandlin, Ph.D.

Clinical Associate Professor

Department of Health and Kinesiology

Texas A&M University, College Station, Texas

"This is a great nutrition primer with a personal touch for the layperson, student, or health educator alike! The information on calcium, vitamins and herbals is especially insightful. The Mix Food Quality Index is a fresh approach to assessing food quality. It should be helpful for all."

Jeffrey L. Lennon, Ph.D., M.D., M.P.H., CHES

Associate Professor of Health Sciences

Liberty University, Lynchburg, Virginia

"A good and informative read. The reference to playing cards is *definitely* relevant to nutrition. While our health is subject to both genetic disposition and lifestyle choices, we now know that we can influence our health risk, even gene expression, through our diet and lifestyle choices. *Play Your Hand Well* reminds us that we are not just subject to the cards we are dealt; instead, you can play your hand well and positively influence, perhaps even ' stack the deck', toward better health, and a long, vibrant life."

Gretchen K. Vannice, MS, RD

Executive Board Member, International Omega-3

Learning and Education Consortium for Health and Medicine

Managing Director, Nutrition Services

Portland, Oregon

"This book covers the essentials of healthy eating and provides a unique tool for choosing healthy foods. Dr. Mix will help you "play the best hand" for a healthy lifestyle."

Michelle Martinez, RD

Health Department

Virginia Beach, Virginia

PLAY
YOUR
HAND WELL

A Nutritional Approach
to Wellness So You Can
Live a Healthier Life Now!

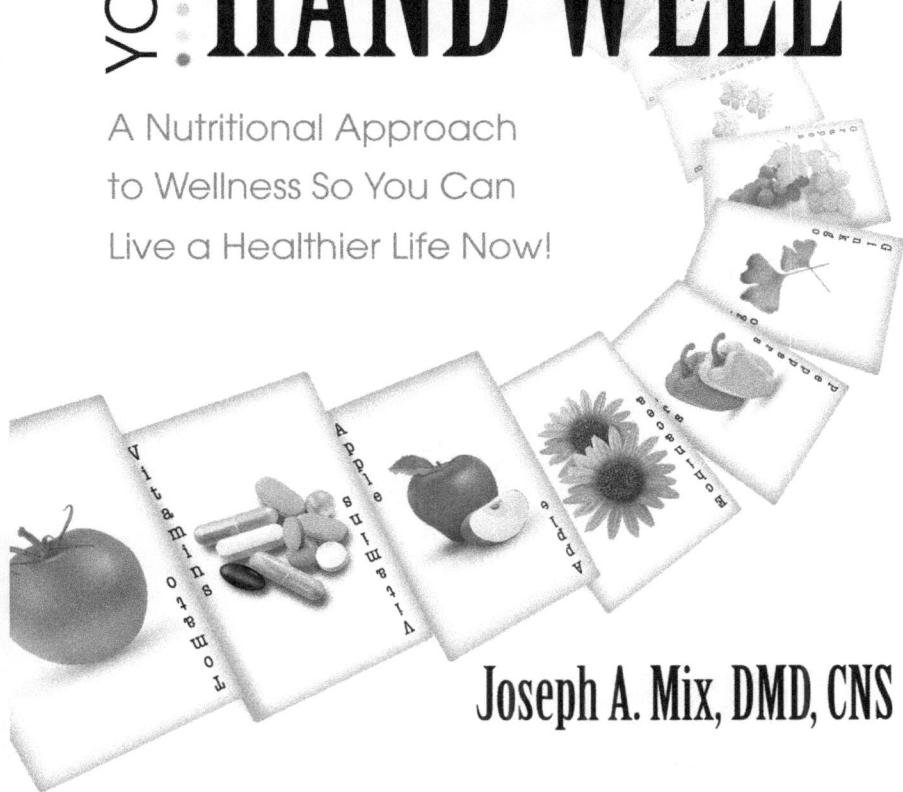

Tomato

Vitamins

Apple Vitamin

Apple

Sunflower

Potatoes

Peppers

Grapes

Ginkgo

Joseph A. Mix, DMD, CNS

LU Books

A Division of Liberty University Press

PLAY YOUR HAND WELL

By Joseph A. Mix, DMD, CNS

ISBN: 978-0-9819357-3-7 (Paperback)

Published by:

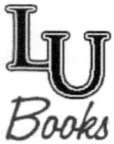

LU Books
A Division of Liberty University Press
Lynchburg, VA

Cover, Interior Designs and Illustrations by:

Megan Johnson
Johnson2Design
www.Johnson2Design.com
megan@Johnson2Design.com

This book is dedicated to Ryan, Becky, and Katie.

ACKNOWLEDGEMENTS

My sincere appreciation goes to my research assistants, Megan Dinsmore and Zach Innocent for their invaluable help in preparing the manuscript, and to my beautiful wife, Lynne, for her constant support, for proofreading the manuscript, and for making Ryan, Becky, and Katie possible.

ABOUT THE AUTHOR
JOSEPH A. MIX, DMD, CNS

Dr. Mix received a Bachelor's degree in Biology from Dickinson College in Carlisle, Pennsylvania and a Doctorate in Dental Medicine from the University of Pittsburgh. He completed a residency in general practice at Langley Air Force Base Hospital in Hampton, Virginia and served as a dentist in the United States Air Force in Aviano, Italy, before entering private practice in New York. He taught operative dentistry at Farleigh Dickinson University in New Jersey and currently is a Professor of Health Sciences at Liberty University in Lynchburg, Virginia.

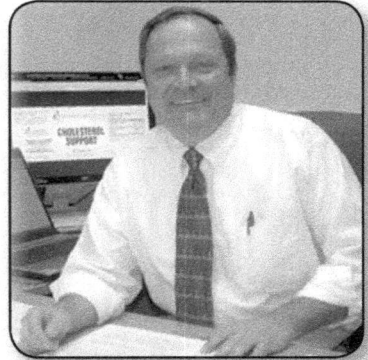

He also holds an adjunct faculty appointment at Virginia Commonwealth University School of Dentistry in Richmond, is a visiting lecturer for the Global Health Program at West Virginia University School of Medicine in Morgantown, and provides dental care for school children in Nelson County through the Virginia Department of Health. Dr. Mix has always been interested in nutrition and issues related to oral health. He is a member of the American College of Nutrition and is a Certified Nutrition Specialist. He has conducted original research in the area of herbal medicine, is published in national peer-reviewed scientific journals, and frequently lectures on health-related topics. He and his wife, Lynne reside in Lynchburg and have 3 children: Ryan, Becky, and Katie.

CONTENTS

INTRODUCTION

It was a cold evening in January and my father was playing a concert in Schenectady, N.Y. He was a consummate musician and recording artist who played on WGY/WRGB Schenectady with his band, *The After Six Seven*. His specialty was the vibraphones, a wonderful melodic instrument that he could caress with four mallets simultaneously and make sing. My mother was home with me; I was 16 months old and asleep in my crib. At intermission, my father felt ill and collapsed in apparent exhaustion. Well-meaning friends, attempting to get him to his feet, struggled with him and carried him to one of the local hospitals across the street where he was pronounced dead on arrival due to a massive heart attack. He was 47.

The dreaded phone call came to my mother: she would now be a single mom, I would have no father, and the heavenly orchestra had just welcomed a new member to its percussion section. That was the day the music died for my mother and me; there would be no more music in our house for the next 18 years. As I grew older, I wondered if I would suffer the same fate as my dad. I am in good health and appreciate the fact that although I cannot change the genetic hand that was dealt me, I can learn to play my hand well and my desire is to help you play your hand well too.

Life is like a card game. You have to play the hand you're dealt. Some people play the game of life better than others. They learn to make the best of their potential and minimize their limitations. As the old song goes: *"You've got to know when to hold 'em and know when to fold 'em..."* You have been dealt a certain set of spiritual and biological possibilities. What you do with them is up to you. You have been given the gift of life and you need to make the most of it. This book can help you live your life to the maximum.

1

This is not a diet book. I've had plenty of opportunities to write diet books over the years but, having attempted various diets myself with rather discouraging results, I'm convinced that a diet book is not the best way to affect long-term behavioral change and impact lives. This is a *lifestyle* book. It is filled with a lifetime of recommendations, tips, suggestions, thoughts and ideas that you will find non-threatening, encouraging, uplifting, and positive. You will also notice that I like to explain the "why." Either it's the teacher in me or my inquisitive mind, but I just can't have someone tell me something, anything, unless he also explains the why to me. You will kindly indulge me as I seek to answer the why throughout this book, which I approach in an easy to read format. In short, my goal is to enable and empower you to live a healthier life now. Though we can't change the cards we've been dealt, it is important to remember that *"every hand's a winner"* and we can learn to play that hand well.

CHAPTER 1
: ALL FATS ARE NOT BAD

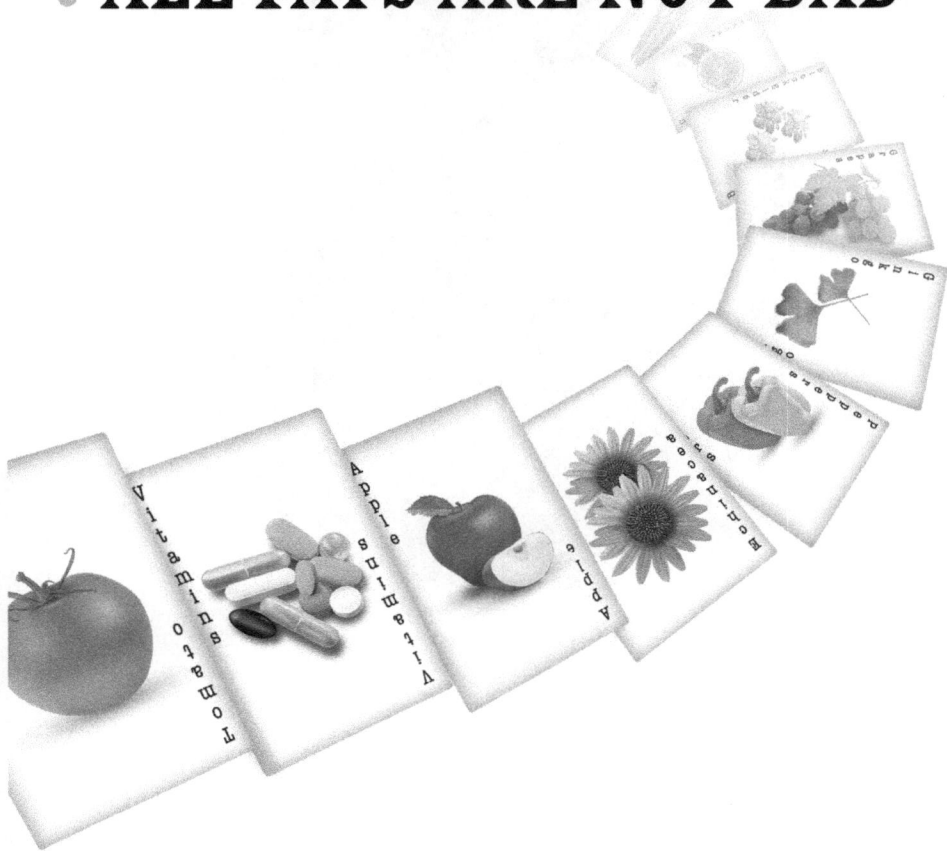

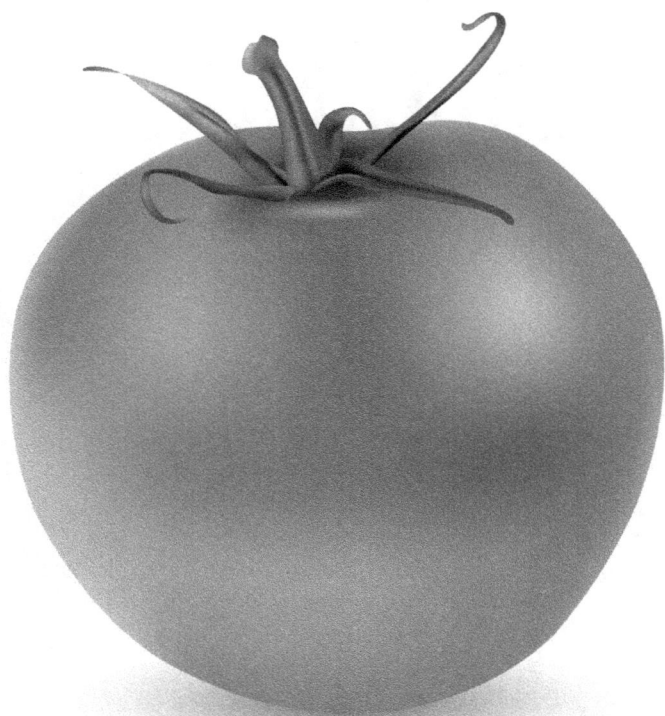

There are so many different diets and nutritional recommendations on the market today, that the average consumer is totally confused. We are told that fat is bad, and that carbohydrates and protein are good. As a result, Americans are eating less fat, more carbohydrates and more protein, yet, obesity, diabetes, heart disease, and cancer are reaching epidemic proportions.[1] Something is not right. Let's take a common sense approach to nutrition, supplementation, diet, and exercise, and see what the research says is "good," what is "bad," and why. By looking at the facts, we can make wise food choices that in turn, lead to healthier, happier and more productive lives.

A Little Chemistry

The body needs fat; there is no doubt whatsoever about that. Fats, also known as *lipids*, are a necessary component of cell membranes and nerves, assist the body with thermal insulation, provide us with a source of energy, and are necessary for the transport and storage of fat-soluble vitamins as well as the formation of cholesterol and steroid hormones. Dietary fat consists mainly of compounds known as *triglycerides*, which are composed of three molecules of fatty acids attached to one molecule of glycerol. The majority of dietary fatty acids vary in length from 4 to 22 carbon atoms in length and may be *saturated* or *unsaturated*. The term *saturation* refers to the degree to which hydrogen atoms attach themselves to the carbon atoms of the fatty acid chain. If each carbon of the fatty acid has its full complement of hydrogen atoms, then the fatty acid is said to be fully saturated. On the other hand, if each carbon atom of the fatty acid chain does *not* possess its full complement of hydrogen atoms and instead forms double bonds with each other, then that fatty acid is said to be *unsaturated*. Unsaturated fatty acids may be either *monounsaturated* (one double bond), or *polyunsaturated* (more than one double bond). Fatty acids are designated by two numbers in parenthesis with the first indicating the number of carbon atoms in the fatty acid chain, and the second, the number of double bonds. Examples of common fatty acids in the diet would be the saturated, *stearic acid* (18:0), the monounsaturated, *oleic acid* (18:1), and the polyunsaturated, *linoleic* (18:2) and *linolenic* (18:3) acids.

Cholesterol: the Good and the Bad

That's enough chemistry for the present time, so let's get right to the point: Because of their respective influences on the cholesterol levels in our blood, *saturated* fats tend to be, well, to put it bluntly, "bad;" monounsaturated fats tend to be rather "good," and polyunsaturated fats are somewhere in between. Let me explain: Cholesterol is a fat, or lipid, that is necessary for life. It is an essential component of all our cell membranes and is necessary to establish proper fluidity and membrane permeability. Though necessary for life, too much cholesterol in the blood is not good. Excess cholesterol in the blood, known as *hypercholesterolemia*, can lead to *atherosclerosis*, clogged and blocked arteries, and, ultimately, a heart attack or stroke. Cholesterol comes from two sources: the diet and the liver and must be transported through the blood, which is largely made up of water. Since fat and water do not mix, the body must provide special carrier molecules known as *lipoproteins* to transport the fatty cholesterol through the watery blood. The two primary lipoproteins responsible for transporting cholesterol are *low-density lipoprotein* (LDL) and *high-density lipoprotein* (HDL). The LDL is easily oxidized (readily combines with unstable oxygen-containing molecules known as *free radicals*). Once oxidized, the LDL is recognized by cells of our immune systems as a foreign invader and an immune response is initiated. The immune response culminates in the formation of *foam cells* (formed by special cells of our immune system, *macrophages*, which eat and engulf the oxidized cholesterol). The foam cell ultimately gets larger and larger until it ruptures and spills its thick, fatty, cholesterol-laden deposits on the inside of the artery wall resulting in an obstruction or fatty *plaque*. The plaque restricts the flow of blood through the artery like a broken down car blocks traffic at a busy intersection. Since the ease at which LDL is oxidized is the central factor in this destructive process, LDL has earned the more common nickname of *"bad cholesterol."* Certain *antioxidant* vitamins, which will be discussed later, can help retard this destructive process and are, therefore, very good.

HDL, on the other hand, acts as a scavenger transporting excess LDL to the liver where it is excreted in the bile. It is protective against heart disease, which is a good thing, and is the reason why HDL is known as *"good cholesterol."* Individual cholesterol levels for HDL and LDL are often used by physicians to assess a patient's risk of developing heart disease. The American Heart Association recommends that your total cholesterol be *below* 200, your LDL be *below* 100, and your HDL should be *above* 40 for men and *above* 50 for women.[2] Many physicians feel that the total cholesterol to HDL *ratio* is a better predictor of overall heart disease risk than either number alone. Ideally, the total cholesterol to HDL ratio should be less than 4.0. I have struggled with my cholesterol much of my adult life. My total cholesterol levels are typically around 240, with my HDL being around 40 and my total to HDL ratio being approximately 6.0. My mother lived to be 89. Her total cholesterol in the year before she died was approximately 300 which would normally have caused alarm had it not been for the fact that her HDL was close to 100 resulting in a total cholesterol to HDL ratio of 3.0! Surprisingly, *dietary* cholesterol does *not* have as significant an impact on the elevation of LDL cholesterol in the blood as dietary saturated fat does. Table 2 summarizes the effects of various dietary factors on the levels of LDL and HDL in the blood.

Saturated Fats

For the most part, with exceptions being *palm* and *coconut* oils, saturated fats are *solid* at room temperature and come from *animal* sources. They, along with *trans-fats*, which will be discussed later, are the two greatest dietary contributors to elevated cholesterol in the blood. The reason that saturated fats (and trans-fats) are so harmful is that they tend to raise the LDL (bad cholesterol), while lowering the HDL (good cholesterol). In addition to elevating the LDL and lowering the HDL, a diet high in saturated fat contributes directly to certain types of cancer, especially breast and colon cancer. In the case of colon cancer, the saturated fat stimulates the release of bile acids, which can be very irritating to the intestine, resulting in an overgrowth of cells produced by the wall of the colon.[3,4] It is well known that *estrogen* (a fat soluble hormone) plays a major role in the development of *breast cancer* and diets high in saturated fat may contribute to this by altering the profile of the sex hormones, thereby facilitating their role in this process.[5] Saturated fats, as already mentioned, are found primarily in products of animal origin, such as milk, cheese, eggs, butter and meat. This also helps explain why vegetarians are less likely to suffer from heart disease, breast or colon cancer.[6] Saturated fat is *not* essential to the diet. While calories from total fat should represent 30% or less of total calories, calories from saturated fat should be kept to a minimum and should comprise no more than 10% of one's daily calorie intake (for an average person on a 2500 calorie per day diet this would mean that no more than 250 of those calories should come from saturated fat, or about 28 grams per day).[7]

Polyunsaturated Fats

When it comes to heart health, the majority of polyunsaturated fats are, for the most part only *"so-so,"* neither greatly beneficial, nor tremendously harmful. These are found primarily in plant oils such as corn, sunflower and safflower oils. They lower the LDL cholesterol, but unfortunately, they also lower the HDL cholesterol. When I first found out that I had elevated cholesterol, and not knowing a great deal about nutrition at the time, I eliminated saturated fat from my diet for six weeks and consumed only polyunsaturated plant oils, thinking that, as those corn oil margarine commercials suggested, I would be doing my heart a big favor. Well, after the six weeks I returned to my doctor for some more blood work and the results were both good and bad. The good news was that my total cholesterol had gone from 280 to 200. The bad news was that my HDL had also gone down, from 46 to 32, so that my total cholesterol to HDL ratio was actually *worse*. If only I had known then what I know now: rather than substituting the saturated fats with the polyunsaturated plant oils, I should have turned to two very good heart-healthy fats which, unfortunately, I knew little about at the time: the omega-3 fats and the monounsaturated fats.

Omega-3 Fats

There is one type of polyunsaturated fat found in soybeans, walnuts, flaxseeds, and fish that are better than so-so; they are good, *very good,* especially for the heart, and are critical for proper neuronal development in infants and children. These are the *omega-3 fats* and are *heart* healthy because they dramatically reduce *triglycerides* in the blood which are also a risk factor for heart disease and, according to the American Heart Association, should be < 150.[2] In addition, they lower the LDL, and possibly raise the HDL cholesterol. Have you ever seen an Eskimo with heart disease? It is rare. Omega-3s first came to our attention many years ago from studies of Eskimos who eat diets high in fatty fish such as tuna, salmon, cod, and mackerel.[8] It was noticed that Eskimos have very low rates of heart disease and further studies found that the omega-3 fats in the fish, specifically DHA and EPA, were the most likely contributing factor. Fish are also a major component of the average *Mediterranean diet* and complement the monounsaturated fats from olive oil quite nicely (see next page). As a result, very low rates of heart disease exist among people living in this geographic region as well. A study reported in the British medical journal *Lancet*, confirmed that eating omega-3 polyunsaturated fats reduced the risk of heart attacks.[9] The heart-protective properties of omega-3 fats are thought to result not only from their ability to lower the LDL and raise the HDL cholesterol, but by several other mechanisms as well: by contributing to the dilation of coronary arteries and thereby reducing the chances of atherosclerosis and a blockage,[10,11] by the prevention of arrhythmias (irregular heartbeats), and by acting as a "blood thinner" and reducing the risk of blood clots.[12,13] In addition to reducing the risk of heart disease, omega-3 contributes to overall health in several other important ways:

- Fish oils demonstrate anti-inflammatory properties and have been recommended in the treatment of arthritis.[14]

- Fish oils are particularly critical to fetal neuronal development.[15]

- Fish oils decrease the symptoms and improves the clinical management of inflammatory bowel disorders such as Crohn's disease and ulcerative colitis.[16]

- Fish oils reduce the risk of certain types of cancer, especially breast and prostate.[17,18]

Monounsaturated Fats

Monounsaturated (one double bond) are also good. The three best sources of monounsaturated oils are, in order, olive oil, canola oil, and peanut oil. Olive oil is the best. My wife and I lived in Italy for three years where we were introduced to its wonderful flavor and multitude of culinary uses and health benefits. If you go to a super market in Italy, you will likely not find corn oil or sunflower oil or safflower oil, but you will find plenty of olive oil and Italians use it copiously. Just as you've probably never met an Eskimo with heart disease, it is likely that you've never met an Italian with heart disease either. Italians have a much lower rate of heart disease compared to Americans, which is likely due to this good fat (and the omega-3 from fish as well). These fats are heart-healthy because they tend to lower the LDL while not lowering the HDL cholesterol (they may even raise the HDL slightly). They also contain vitamin E, an antioxidant that helps protect cell membranes and has demonstrated heart-healthy properties. Folks who live in the Mediterranean region have known this for quite some time because 50% of their daily fat intake comes from olive oil.[19] Olive oil can be used for all types of cooking and can be used cold on salads, vegetables, and snacks. My family enjoys making popcorn in an air popper and then, rather than saturating it with butter, we pour on a little olive oil for a delightfully tasty and healthy snack. Additionally, I was told of a woman who lowered her total cholesterol simply by combining olive oil, half and half, with butter. She made her own "spread" and when used in moderation in place of regular butter or margarine, the olive oil was able to lower her LDL by about 20 points.

Partially Hydrogenated Fats

Before leaving the topic of fats in the diet, there is one other type of fat that requires discussion: *partially hydrogenated fats*. Partially hydrogenated fats are made from polyunsaturated vegetable oils such as corn, sunflower, safflower and soybean oils through a process known as *hydrogenation*. The process began in the 1960s as a low cost alternative to saturated animal fats and became commonly used in deep-fat frying, baking and margarine spreads. Hydrogenation involves exposing hydrogen to the polyunsaturated plant oils, which are in liquid form, and, as you will remember, have more than one double bond. Exposure to hydrogen breaks some of these double bonds and the plant oil becomes less *unsaturated* and more *saturated*. As it does, it is converted from a liquid into a semi-solid, which is more "spreadable." The hydrogenation process, however, creates abnormal molecules known as *trans-fatty acids*, which have been linked to both heart disease and cancer in laboratory animals and humans.[20] Trans-fats are bad, very bad, since they act similarly to the saturated fats in that they raise the LDL (bad) cholesterol and lower the HDL (good) cholesterol.[21] In fact, some studies indicate that the trans fatty acids are actually *worse* than the saturated fats and have the most unfavorable effects on blood lipids of all dietary fatty acids. The LDL to HDL cholesterol ratio with a trans fatty acid-enriched diet is nearly double that of a diet with an equivalent amount of saturated fat.[22] While neither would be considered a healthy food, if you were to ask me to choose between butter and margarine, because of the trans-fat connection, I would have to choose the butter. Butter does contain saturated fats and, therefore, should be used sparingly. A healthier alternative to margarine may be found by mixing butter half and half with olive oil as mentioned earlier. This makes a tasty, healthy spread free of hydrogenated fats and may actually lower cholesterol when used in moderation as a substitute for margarine.

You have just had a primer in fats. You now know the good fats, the bad fats, and the ones in between. If I could make three recommendations, it would be to *decrease* your intake of saturated fat, *eliminate* your intake of trans-fats, and *increase* the amounts of both olive oil and fish oil in your diet. As we have seen, the beneficial effects of these two fats alone are tremendous (for those who do not care to eat fish, fish oil may be purchased in capsules and taken up to three times daily as directed). Now let's look at another important class of nutrients: the carbohydrates. You are beginning to play your hand well!

CHAPTER 2
: ALL CARBOHYDRATES ARE NOT GOOD

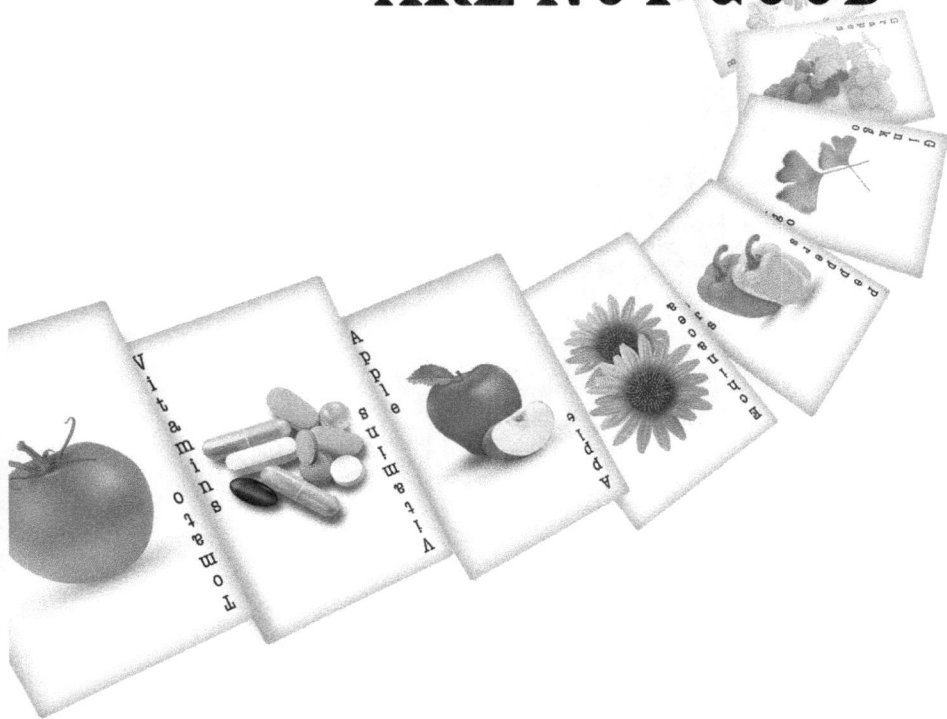

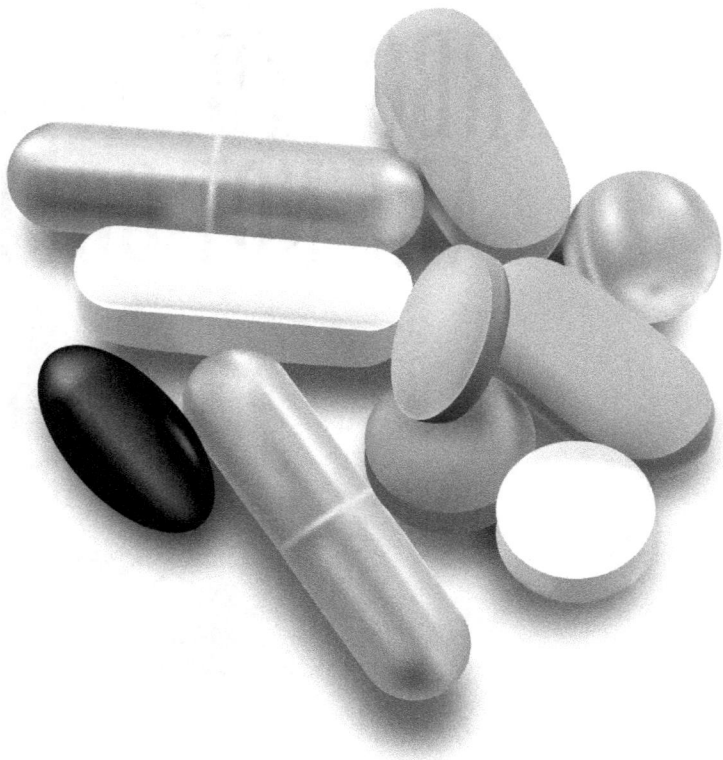

C arbohydrates exist as molecules of sugar bound together in chains of varying lengths. Long chains of sugar molecules bound together (starch and fiber, for examples) are known as *complex* carbohydrates or polysaccharides, while the *simple* carbohydrates merely consist of single sugar molecules (monosaccharides), or double sugar molecules (disaccharides) and are not bound together as long chains. Most carbohydrates are *digestible*, which refers to their ability to be broken down by the digestive system and absorbed into the bloodstream where they become an available source of energy for the cells of the body. Fiber, a complex carbohydrate, is *indigestible* to humans, but nevertheless, possesses many health benefits that will be discussed shortly.

Good Carbs and Bad Carbs

Generally speaking, from a dietary standpoint, simple carbohydrates are "bad" and complex carbohydrates are, for the most part, "good." Let me explain why: the simple carbohydrates (sugars) are bad because they require little digestion, are absorbed into the bloodstream very rapidly, thereby causing a sudden, dramatic increase in blood sugar. This sudden increase in blood sugar, in turn, causes the pancreas to release rather large amounts of the hormone *insulin* that rapidly lowers blood sugar, sometimes to dangerously low levels. Diets high in simple carbohydrates cause this cycle to be repeated many times throughout the day and this high blood sugar/low blood sugar roller-coaster often leads to severe hunger cravings, fat storage, mood swings, and diabetes. Complex carbohydrates on the other hand, must be digested, which takes both time and energy, and therefore do not cause such a pronounced, rapid rise in blood sugar.

The "Glycemic" Response

The rate at which a particular food elicits a rise in blood glucose is called the *"glycemic response,"* and foods that cause a rapid rise in blood sugar, are said to have a high glycemic response.[1] The glycemic response of a particular food is measured by comparing the rate at which it elicits a rise in blood glucose relative to pure glucose. This measure is known as the glycemic index and is very useful in making wise food choices. Pure glucose has a glycemic index of 100 and all other foods are relative to it. Foods that have a high glycemic index are mainly the simple sugars, but also include some starches and baked goods made from processed, refined, white flour.[2] High glycemic index foods result in high insulin levels, elicited by the rapid rise in blood sugar. In time, high levels of insulin not only lead to fat storage and obesity, but also to pancreatic "burnout" and diabetes.[3] In the last 15 years the average American has reduced his fat intake from 41% to 34%, yet has gained eight pounds which is largely attributable to over-consumption of carbohydrates made from refined, processed flour and sugar. More alarming, obesity among children has doubled in the last two decades, and diabetes has reached epidemic proportions among many populations over the same time period.[4]

Healthier alternatives to these processed, refined, high glycemic index simple carbohydrates are the complex carbohydrates. Complex carbohydrates are found in fresh fruits and vegetables, whole grains, and nuts. These carbohydrates are good because they elicit a slower, less pronounced rise in blood sugar and have a *lower* "glycemic index." With a slower rise in blood sugar, less insulin is released, and consequently, the tendencies for hunger cravings, fat storage and diabetes are lower. The glycemic index for selected foods is given in Table 1. The glycemic response (and its corresponding insulin response) can be modulated (slowed down) by three things in the diet: fat, fiber, and protein. As it is not always possible to eliminate high glycemic index foods from the diet, combining them with fat, fiber, and/or protein will slow the release of glucose into the bloodstream.

Fiber

Fiber, what your grandmother called "roughage," is an example of a complex carbohydrate with excellent health benefits:

- Fiber lowers the risk of colon cancer by diluting the contents of the colon and protecting it from the hazardous material found in fecal waste (bile acids, etc). It also stimulates *peristalsis*, the rhythmic contraction of the bowel as it propels waste, thereby reducing transit time (the time it takes for waste to clear the colon). The less time the waste stays in the colon, the less contact it has with the colon wall, the less chance of irritation, and the less opportunity for initiating a pre-cancerous lesion.

- Fiber lowers cholesterol. Some of the medications used today to lower cholesterol are classified as "bile-sequestering agents" and work the same way as fiber. Fiber combines with bile which is an emulsifier produced by the liver and stored by the gallbladder. Bile is largely made up of cholesterol and it assists in the digestion of fat. The bile emulsifies the fat the same way that your dish detergent breaks up the big globs of fat and grease on your cooking utensils so that they can be dissolved in water and rinsed down the drain. Bile is recycled by the body and used over and over. By combining with the bile, the fiber prevents the bile from being recycled and forces the body to manufacture more bile instead. Since bile is largely made up of cholesterol, the liver must take cholesterol from the blood to make the bile, with the end result being that the level of cholesterol in the blood goes down.

- Fiber lowers the risk of *diverticulitis*. Diverticulitis is the most common gastrointestinal disease of persons over age 40. It is a weakening in the wall of the colon caused by eating soft, canned and processed foods that are low in fiber, resulting in pouches or *diverticuli* which periodically get infected and cause great distress. Diverticulitis is almost non-existent in developing countries where high fiber diets are more prevalent. Fiber provides bulk in the stool, which offers resistance to the muscular wall of the colon thereby strengthening it and preventing these diverticuli from forming in the first place.

- Fiber helps to prevent hemorrhoids. Hemorrhoids are varicose veins in the anal region, which are largely the result of constipation. Straining during bowel movements impedes the blood flow and the veins become swollen and inflamed (hemorrhoids). By promoting peristalsis, the movement of fecal waste through the bowel is facilitated, constipation is relieved, and the chance of hemorrhoids is greatly lessened.

- Fiber, as mentioned above, slows the rise in blood sugar.

- Fiber assists us with calorie control by helping us to feel "full" so we don't overeat.[5,6] (Admit it: when you tried the Atkin's diet, did you ever really feel full?)

In the past, dietary fiber was classified as soluble or insoluble based on its ability to dissolve in water. Insoluble fiber was generally thought to produce bulking of the stool and that soluble fiber lowered cholesterol. It is now known that certain types of soluble fiber can increase stool weight as effectively as insoluble fiber. Similarly, not all soluble fiber is capable of lowering cholesterol, so it has been recommended that the former classification be discontinued.[7]

The best sources of fiber are raw fruits and vegetables, whole grains, and bran. Whole grains include the *entire* grain which is comprised of four parts: the *husk or chaff* which has no nutritional value, the *endosperm* comprised largely of starch that provides nourishment for the developing *germ*, the *germ* that will develop into a new plant and is a great source of vitamin E, and the *bran*, which is an excellent source of fiber and B vitamins. Unfortunately, when grains are processed and converted into refined, bleached, white flour, much of the nourishment is lost. The refining process eliminates the germ and the bran and leaves only the endosperm, which is rapidly converted, into glucose upon ingestion (high glycemic index). Since whole grains contain all parts of the grain, the fat from the germ and the fiber from the bran combine to make the glycemic response of the endosperm much *lower* than would be the case from refined grain products. Italians have long recognized this: they love their fish, and they love their olive oil, but they also love their whole grain pasta! Try it sometime; you may even wish to experiment with using whole grain flour for all or most of your baking. As an added benefit, the complex carbohydrates found in fresh fruits and vegetables, whole grains and nuts contain large amounts of vitamins and minerals, such as potassium, magnesium, calcium, folic acid, and B vitamins.[8] Juice, by the way, has little, if any fiber, is very high in sugar and possesses a high glycemic index. It is mostly all calories and for calorie control it is better to eat the whole fruit than to drink the juice made from it. Don't drink your calories! This applies to high fructose corn syrup (HFCS). Try to stay away from this if at all possible; more empty calories and a precursor to obesity.

What About Those "No-Carb" and "Low-Carb" Diets?

Approximately 60% of a person's daily calories should come from carbohydrates (see Figure 2 on Page 30). Carbohydrates from fresh fruits and vegetables should form the basis of a healthy diet. It is good to eliminate the *bad* carbs (simple sugars, foods made from processed, white flour, those with a high glycemic index) but it is certainly not good to eliminate *all* carbohydrates. The theory behind the "no-carb" and "low-carb" diets that are popular today is that they prevent elevations of insulin and encourage lipolysis (fat burning). Initially, there is considerable weight loss (much of it water), but it comes at a price:

- In the absence of carbohydrate, fat will be incompletely oxidized (burned) and will form compounds known as ketones. *Ketosis* occurs which throws the delicate acid/base balance of the body out of kilter. This puts a strain on the liver and kidneys and causes a compensatory urinary calcium loss resulting in weakened bones.[9]

- You have to get your calories somewhere and the only options are carbs, fats, and protein. Now if you are not consuming carbs, then most likely you will be consuming too much saturated fat and protein, which exacerbates (makes worse) your acid/base imbalance, your urinary calcium loss, and the strain on your kidneys and liver.

- Alternatively, low-carb diets lead to an insufficiency of certain vitamins, minerals and fiber.[10]

In summary then, select foods that have a *low* glycemic index; choose pasta and baked goods made from *whole* grain flour; eat sweet potatoes (a great source of complex carbs, fiber, and the anti-oxidant vitamin, beta-carotene) instead of white potatoes (all starch); limit juice; and eat lots of fresh fruits and vegetables (raw 50% of the time), whole grains, and nuts. Your hand is looking better and better!

Table 1. The Glycemic Index.

EAT LESS		EAT MORE	
Food	**Glycemic Index**	**Food**	**Glycemic Index**
Sugars		*Sugars*	
• Glucose	100	• Honey	87
Vegetables		*Vegetables*	
• Parsnips	98	• Soybeans	15
• Carrots	90	• Kidney beans	30
• White potatoes	70	• Lentils	25
		• Sweet potatoes	48
Fruit		*Fruit*	
• Bananas	65	• Apples	36
• Raisins	68	• Oranges	40
Grains		*Grains*	
• White flour spaghetti	56	• Whole wheat spaghetti	40
• Cornflakes	85	• Oats	48
• White rice	70	• Brown rice	60
• White flour pancakes	66	• Buckwheat pancakes	45
• White bread	76	• Whole wheat bread	64

CHAPTER 3
: IF PROTEIN IS GOOD, IS MORE BETTER?

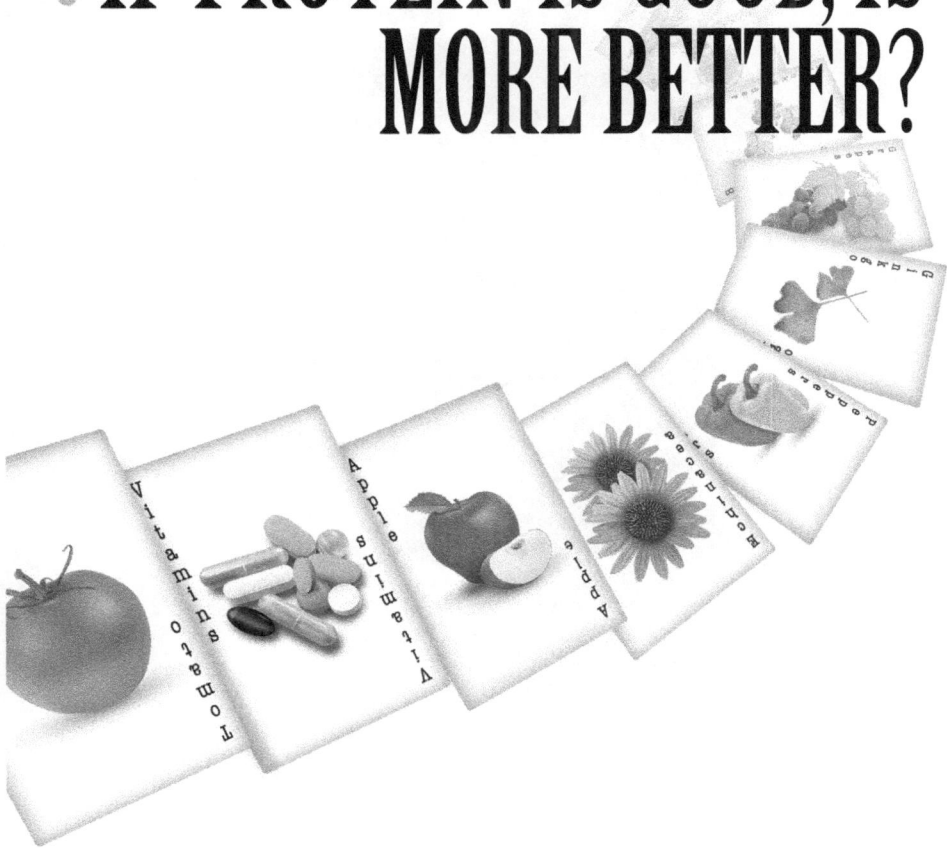

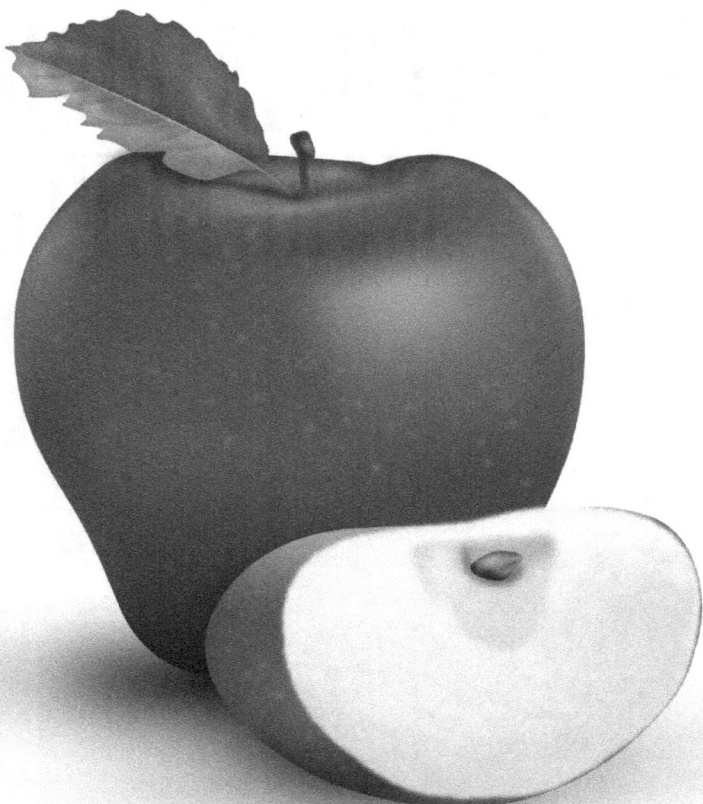

Protein is made up of individual units known as *amino acids*, which are the bricks or building blocks of the body. Protein is found in plants, especially legumes, and in animals. Most Americans consume the majority of their dietary protein from meat as well as other animal products including milk, eggs and cheese. Proteins are the bricks and mortar of the body. They make up most of the physical body, including muscles, bones, ligaments, tendons, antibodies (chemical substances of the immune system), neurotransmitters of the nervous system, regulatory hormones, enzymes, and specialized carrier molecules such as hemoglobin. The turnover rate for many of these proteins is high and they continually need to be dismantled and rebuilt. Proteins are made up of 20 or so different amino acids, which constitute the "complete set" required for the body to synthesize a particular protein. The "blueprint" for the synthesis of a particular protein is encoded in the cell's DNA. Each protein requires a different combination of amino acids. If some of the bricks (amino acids) are missing, a protein will not be built, and the body suffers. *Animal* protein (milk, eggs, fish, poultry, beef) contains all of the essential amino acids necessary for protein construction and, therefore, is of "high quality." High quality protein is especially important for those stages of life and activities that are characterized by building muscle, i.e., infancy, childhood, pregnancy, and athletics. The unfortunate thing about animal protein, however, is that it usually contains large amounts of saturated fat—the *bad* fat. We know that folks who consume diets high in meat are at a greater risk of heart disease and cancer, due largely in part, to the high saturated fat content, but perhaps due to other factors as well.

Extremely high protein diets (> 30% of daily caloric intake) put a tremendous strain on the liver and the kidney (the liver, because it has to remove the nitrogen from protein, and the kidney because it has to eliminate the nitrogen from the body in the urine). Diets high in protein also present other health problems; including, osteoporosis, kidney stones, and dehydration.[1] Permit me to offer a rather brief and simplistic, yet useful, explanation as to the link between high intakes from animal protein and these diseases:

The amino acids that comprise protein, unlike fats and carbohydrates, are not stored to any great degree by the body. They are used to build a protein, stored as fat, or are dismantled and eliminated in the urine. Breaking down protein to individual amino acids is accomplished by a process known as *hydrolysis*, which requires water; hence, dehydration is often seen in people who are on high protein diets. Circulating large amounts of amino acids in the blood creates an acid environment characterized by a low blood pH, a condition known as *acidosis*. In the same way that farmers use lime (calcium carbonate) to neutralize acid soils, and those with heartburn use Tums® or Rolaids® (calcium carbonate) to neutralize acid reflux, so, too, the result of acidosis is that calcium is employed by the body to restore neutrality. Where does the calcium come from? You guessed it, the bones! Large amounts of calcium being pulled from the bones and participating in a buffering system to neutralize the blood will lead to elevated levels of calcium in the urine (hypercalciuria) and may also lead not only to osteoporosis, but also to kidney stones.[2,3] Some animal protein in the diet is perfectly fine, but diets high in animal protein are not good (the reason that the high protein diets *do* result in weight loss is due to a lowered insulin response from the pancreas as compared to the insulin response from carbohydrates, *and* from the large amounts of water lost by the body in the metabolism of the protein).

Plant Protein

Plant protein, on the other hand, does *not* seem to be associated with these deleterious health concerns. Plant protein is found in grains, legumes, seeds and

PLAY YOUR HAND WELL

nuts. Unfortunately, plant protein is not of such high quality as animal protein. That means that any single plant, with the exception of the *soybean*, probably does *not* contain all the essential amino acids needed for protein building. To provide all the essential amino acids, the vegetarian diet must include on a daily basis food from each of the above categories: grains, legumes, *and* seeds and nuts, in order to be considered complete.[4]

How much protein is the right amount? The adult RDA for protein is 0.8 grams per kg body weight per day. This seems to be about right. Much more than this, especially from animal sources, would likely contribute to some of the health problems we talked about earlier. A 60 kg woman (132 lbs.) should consume approximately 50 grams of protein per day, which, at 4 calories per gram, would account for 10-15% of her daily caloric intake. Should she be an athlete, her additional daily protein requirement would be half again as much. With at least half of her total daily protein coming from *plant* protein, (grains, legumes, *and* seeds and nuts), she is well on her way to a healthy, happy, productive, physically fit life. Carbohydrate-sensitive individuals who gain weight at the drop of a hat on high carbohydrate diets, people with hypoglycemia (low blood sugar), and diabetics may find it helpful to increase the percentage of protein in the diet from 10-15% to 20-25 % of total calories. Protein modulates the insulin response, which tends to keep the blood sugar levels on an even keel, resulting in less tendency toward hunger cravings, hypoglycemia and fat storage. It should be emphasized again that the super-high protein diets, along with protein and amino acid *supplementation* are *not* necessary and may lead to some of the problems discussed earlier.

Table 2. Effects of Various Dietary Factors on Blood Levels of LDL and HDL Cholesterol.

DIETARY FACTOR	LDL (Bad)	HDL (Good)
Saturated Fat	increases	decreases
Cholesterol	little effect	little effect
Polyunsaturated Fat	decreases	decreases
Monounsaturated Fat	decreases	may increase slightly
Omega-3	decreases	may increase slightly
Fiber	decreases	little effect
High Caloric Intake	increases	decreases
Trans Fatty Acids	increases	decreases
Protein	little effect	little effect
Simple Carbohydrates (sugar)	increases	little effect
Complex Carbohydrates (starches)	little effect	little effect

PLAY YOUR HAND WELL

Homocysteine

Motivated by my Dad's premature death, and wondering what hand I had been dealt, I read everything I could find on the subject of heart disease. When, back in the 1990s, it was determined that elevated levels of the amino acid *homocysteine* increased the risk of coronary artery disease, I wanted do conduct research to learn more.

After much research (which consisted of a rather extensive review of the literature), I learned that there was indeed a connection between elevated levels of homocysteine in the blood and heart disease, but I also learned that there was a very simple, inexpensive and safe way to keep these levels in check: *folic acid*. 1 mg of folic acid per day, from food and/or supplement form, can effectively lower elevated homocysteine levels, thereby reducing the risk of heart disease. I learned that folic acid works with vitamin B_{12} to reduce homocysteine levels and I also found what apparently other researchers had missed: the fact that large doses of vitamin C (500 mg-1000 mg) may interfere with folic acid's ability to lower elevated homocysteine levels.[5]

The bottom line here is that yes, indeed homocysteine is another risk factor that you need to know about. It is nothing to worry about, but you need to know. Have your homocysteine levels checked by your physician. Normal levels are between 5 and 15 micromoles per liter with levels over 15 considered elevated. Should your homocysteine levels be elevated, do the following:

- Increase the amounts of fresh fruits and vegetables in your diet, which are good sources of folic acid.
- Do not take more than 500 mg of vitamin C per day in supplement form.
- Take a dietary supplement of folic acid.

Figure 2. Composition of the Ideal Diet.

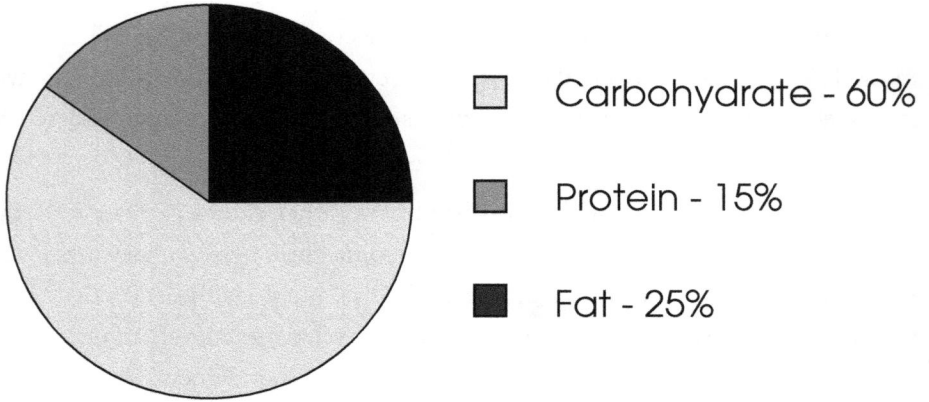

☐ Carbohydrate - 60%

▨ Protein - 15%

■ Fat - 25%

CHAPTER 4
: BREAKFAST IS GOOD

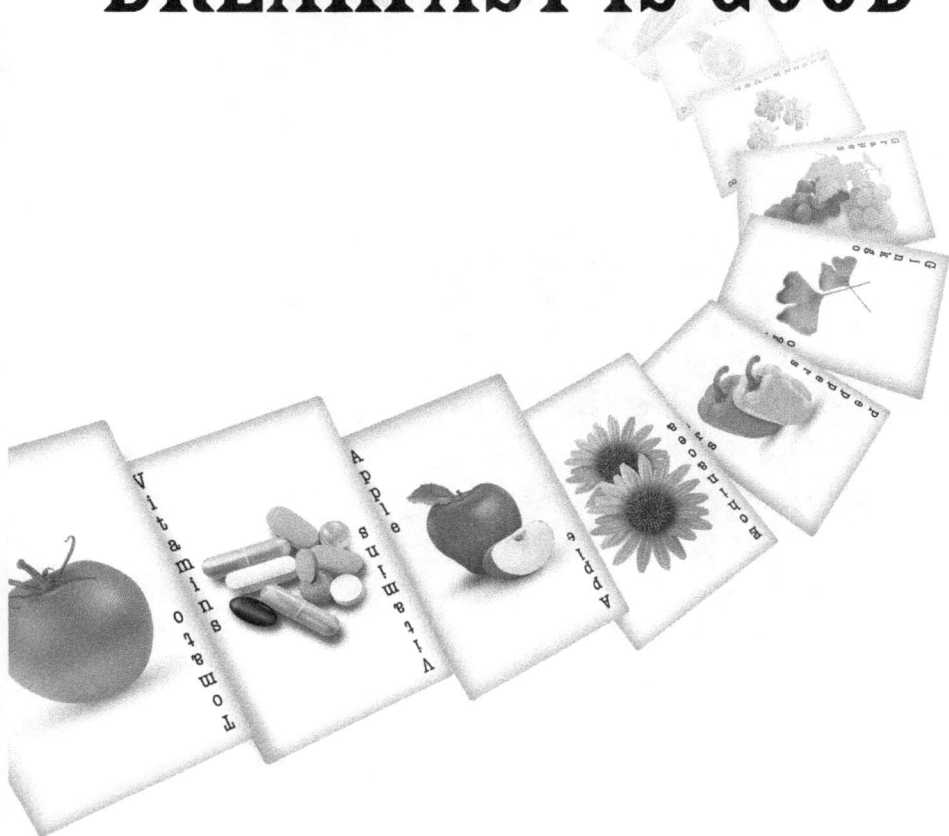

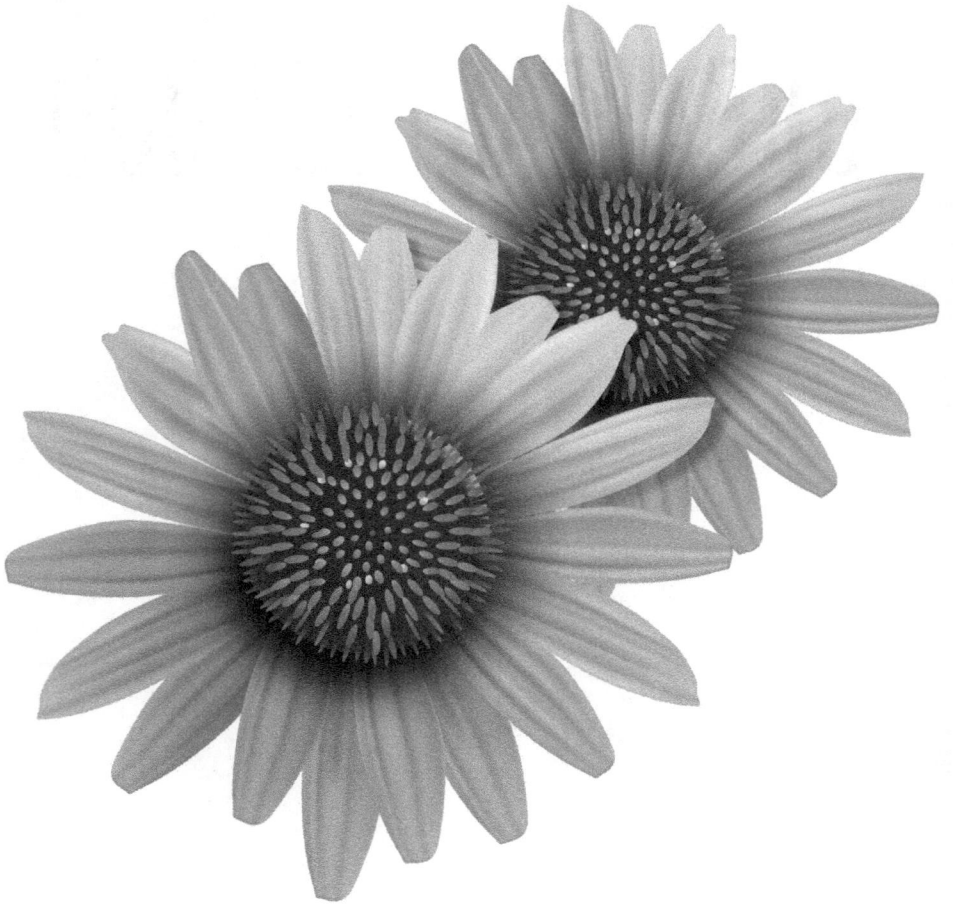

Figure 3. Breakfast: a Great Way to Start the Day Off Right!

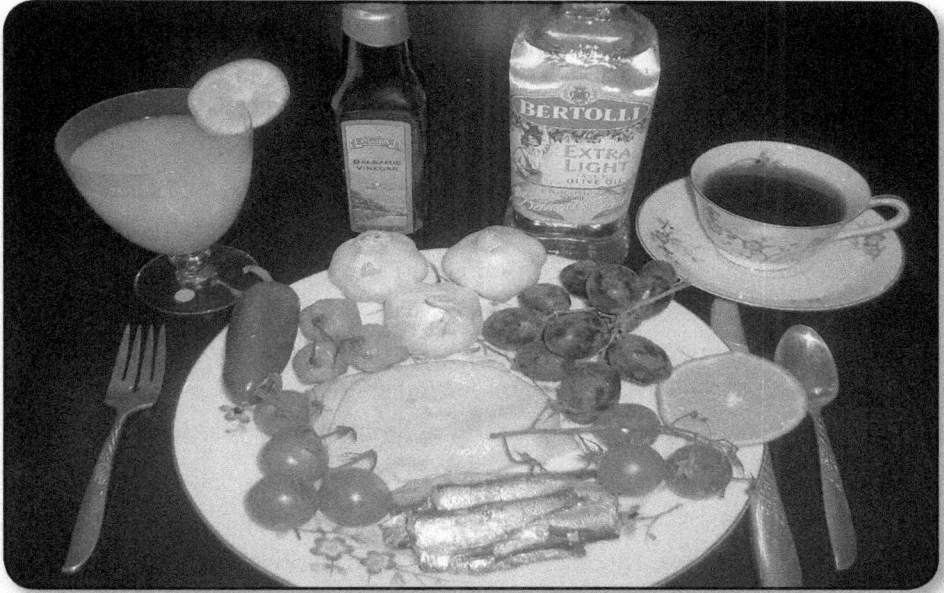

Sadly, only about 50% of Americans eat breakfast regularly. This is unfortunate because breakfast is good. We know that students who eat a nutritious breakfast perform better in school and we know that people who consume a large percentage of their daily caloric intake early in the day are less obese and have fewer nutrition-related health problems than those who skip breakfast. Let us revisit the Mediterranean diet. As I mentioned earlier, my wife and I lived in Italy for three years and during those three years we watched what the Italians ate. Believe me, Italians know how to eat a good breakfast! The typical American breakfast consists of cereal, toast, juice, and perhaps a bagel. Each of these foods possesses a very high glycemic index. Having just gotten out of bed, this breakfast presents quite a "jolt to the system" by increasing blood sugar levels so quickly and dramatically that the equally-dramatic insulin response which follows starts the high blood sugar/low blood sugar roller-coaster. Blood sugar is driven down by the large insulin response, and by 10:00 a.m., the average American is starving. Mediterranean people, on the other hand consume breakfasts of fresh fruit and vegetables that are high in fiber, and protein (usually fish, sometimes turkey, chicken, or veal).[1] This diet does not cause the blood sugar to rise so abruptly; the insulin response is not as pronounced, and blood sugar levels remain on an even keel which helps to stave off hunger until noon or after. Figure 4 compares hypothetical blood glucose values for persons consuming a typical American versus Mediterranean breakfast. Assuming the breakfast is consumed at 8:00 AM shortly after each wakes up, and assuming that each person begins with a fasting blood glucose value of 70, note the higher peaks and valleys from the high carbohydrate American breakfast compared to the lower glycemic index Mediterranean diet. The rapid rises seen in the American breakfast are followed by sharp declines as a result of the insulin response.

Another benefit to be derived from breakfast is that it tends to raise metabolism (the BMR or Basal Metabolic Rate). It takes calories to burn calories and consuming a healthy breakfast raises your thermostat a tad bit higher so that you will continue to burn more calories throughout the day. By contrast, those who do not consume breakfast go into what is known as a "starvation mode" which causes the body to set its thermostat lower in order to conserve calories, rather than burn them. Many researchers feel that calories consumed early in the day tend to get burned or utilized, while calories consumed later tend to get stored as fat. As a rule of thumb, it is not wise to eat within four hours of going to bed, since most of these calories will not be "burned off" and will end up in fat storage.

Figure 4. Hypothetical Blood Glucose Levels for Persons Consuming a Typical American Versus Mediterranean Breakfast.

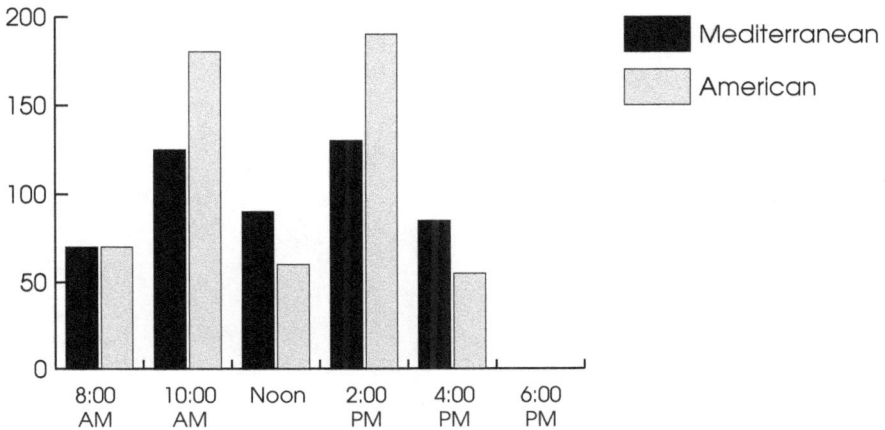

As mentioned earlier, breakfast is a great opportunity to start your day off right. Fresh fruits and vegetables and protein from lean meat help to keep your blood sugar and insulin levels down. Fish is great for breakfast. Not only do you get omega-3 fats, but tuna, for example, is an excellent source of the amino acid, *tyrosine*. Tyrosine is an important component of *neurotransmitters* (brain chemicals), such as *dopamine*, *norepinephrine*, and *epinephrine*. Thyroid hormones also require tyrosine. Epinephrine, also known as *adrenaline*, is a very powerful stimulant and the mediator of the "fight or flight" response that results in an energy rush. You may wish to try tuna for breakfast and see if it doesn't provide you with a bit more energy in the morning!

CHAPTER 5
WATER IS GOOD

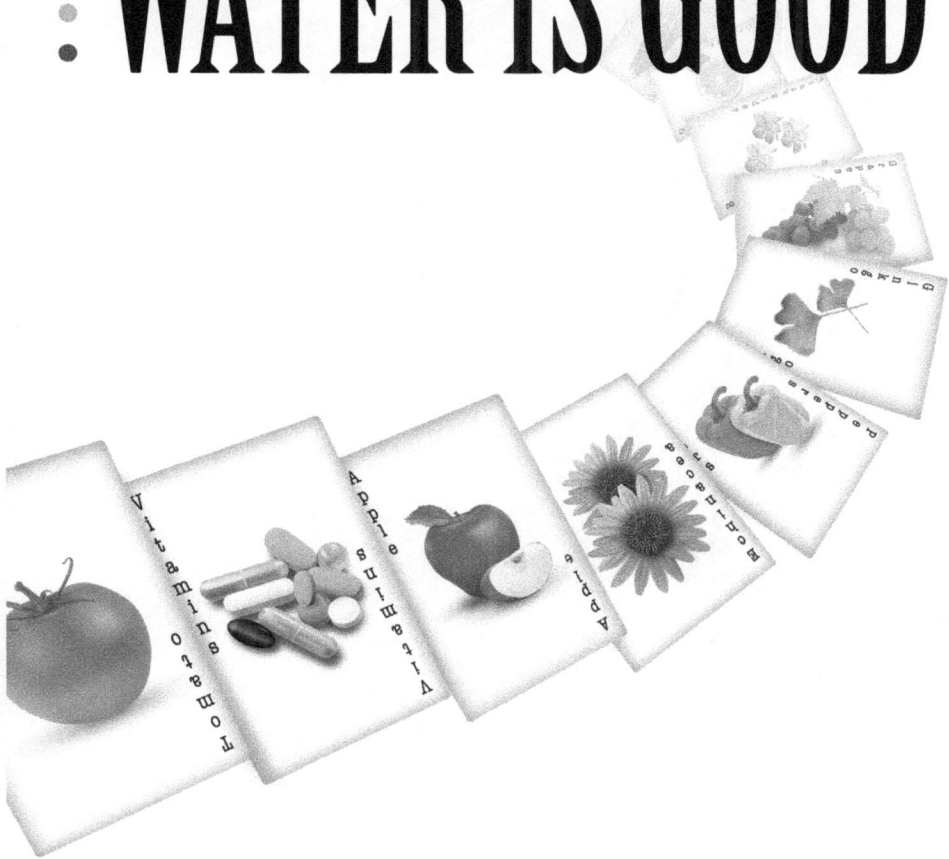

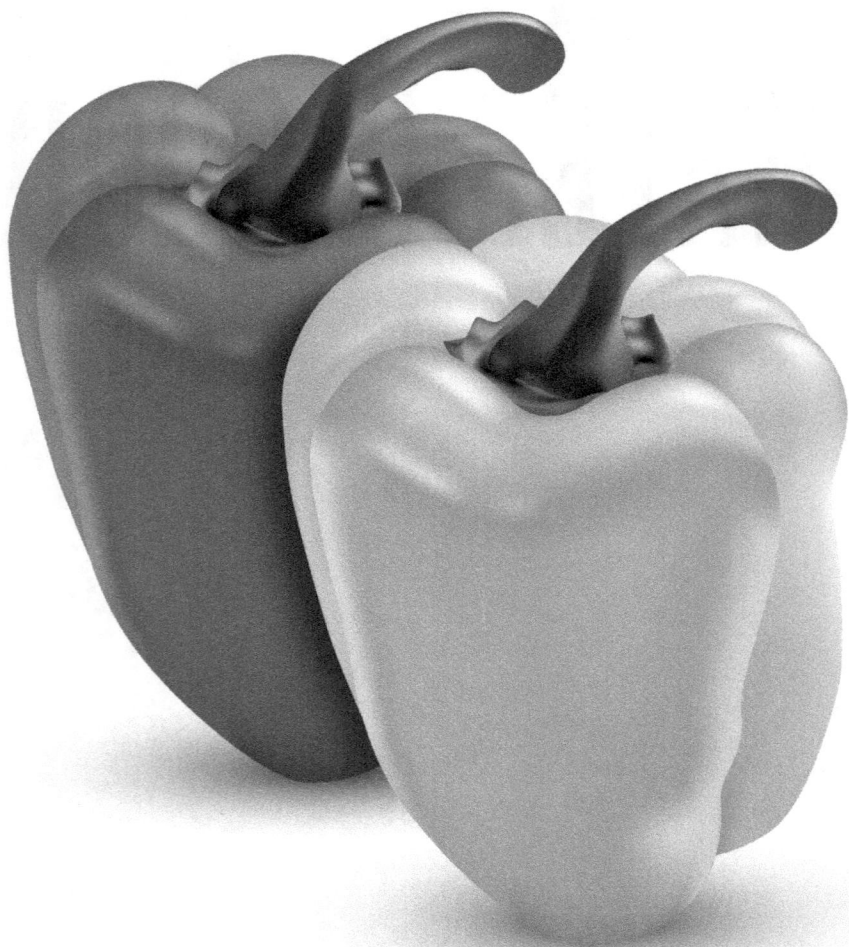

Figure 5. Water is Essential for Life and Critical for Our Existence.

"Water is the physiological river upon which vital nutrients navigate the pathways of metabolism. Without water, all other nutrients are as parched silt and sand at the bottom of a dry river bed."[1]

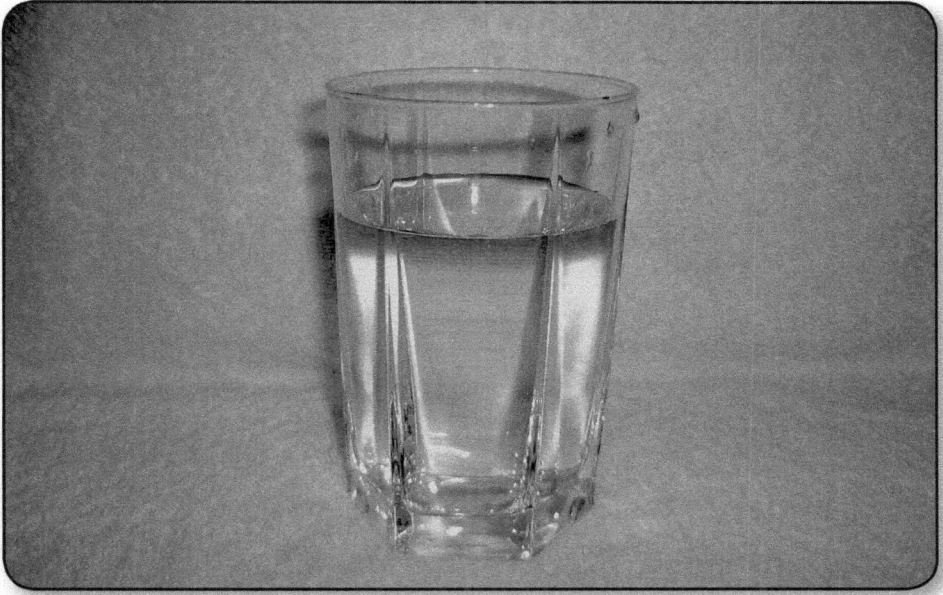

W ater is so important and the average American is probably dehydrated most of the time and consumes far less than the recommended six to eight glasses per day. Drink water, lots of water. Drink it with meals in place of a high-caloric beverage. The *hypothalamus* gland, located in the brain, governs thirst and tells you when you need to drink. This thirst mechanism lags behind your actual need for water so that by the time you feel thirsty, you are most likely already dehydrated. Keep well hydrated throughout the entire day; your body requires about 1 milliliter per calorie spent per day. For an average person who spends approximately 2000 calories per day, this would be equal to 2000 milliliters or two liters per day (approximately two quarts per day or eight glasses of water per day). More is required for pregnancy, lactation, and athletic activity.

Sources of water to meet the body's needs come from drinking water and other beverages, foods, and metabolic byproducts as shown in Figure 6.

Figure 6. Sources of Drinking Water.

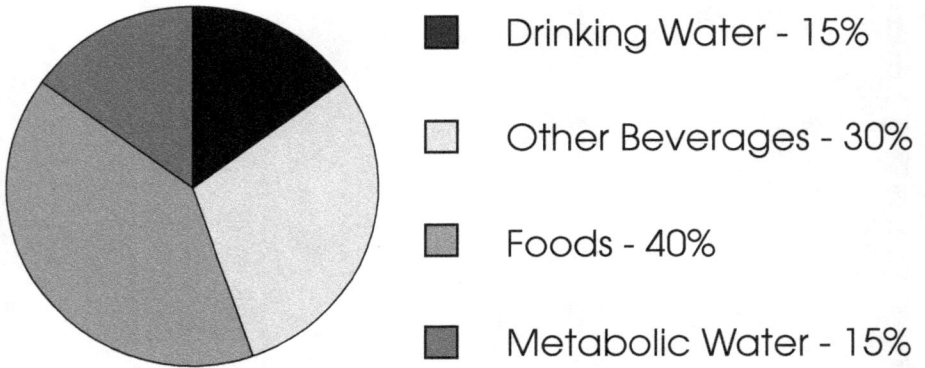

- ■ Drinking Water - 15%
- ☐ Other Beverages - 30%
- ■ Foods - 40%
- ■ Metabolic Water - 15%

By weight, water makes up about 60% of the human male body and 50-55% of the female body, which has a higher proportion of fat. The water content of various organs ranges from 83% in the blood to 10% in adipose (fat) tissue. Water is distributed throughout the body, but is found primarily in two compartments, one within cells (intracellular) and one between cells the (extracellular). Extracellular water includes fluid located between tissues (interstitial) and in the blood plasma. Water plays a key role in maintaining *homeostasis* (the tendency of the body to maintain a stable internal environment), provides a medium for transport of nutrients and the elimination of wastes, allows biochemical reactions such as digestion and energy production to take place, provides for protection in the form of tears, spinal fluid and amniotic fluid, and is crucial to the body's ability to get rid of excess heat by the evaporation of sweat.

Dehydration decreases the core body temperature and contributes to electrolyte loss, both of which can dramatically decrease exercise performance. *Rehydration* is very important and especially when engaging in athletic exercise; the athlete should begin his/her activity in a hydrated state and continue to drink water throughout to compensate for fluid losses from sweat which differ for various sports as seen in Table 3. Table 4 provides a recipe for making your own oral rehydration solution.

Table 3. Sweating Rates for Different Sports[2]

Sport	Liters Per Hour	
	Mean	Range
Water Polo	0.55	0.30 – 0.80
Cycling	0.80	0.29 – 1.25
Running	1.10	0.54 – 1.83
Basketball	1.11	0.70 – 1.60
Soccer	1.17	0.70 – 2.10

In addition to excessive sweating, dehydration can also be caused by the following:

● Insufficient water intake

● Medications such as diuretics which are used to lower blood pressure

- Caffeine
- Excessive sodium consumption
- Excessive protein intake (see Chapter 3)
- High fiber diet

Water can be obtained from a well, from a municipal supply, a tap or a bottle. Have it analyzed by sending it off to your local health department or a lab equipped to perform reliable water analysis. What we refer to as *"hard water,"* may actually be quite good for you. By "hard" we mean that it contains relatively *high* amounts of various minerals such as calcium and magnesium. You will notice that "hard" water does not lather or bubble up as nicely as "soft" water and it may leave a ring around your tub and sink. If this is a problem, then you may wish to have a water filtration system installed, which bypasses the main tap from which you get your drinking water. *"Soft"* water tends to be *low* in calcium and magnesium and *high* in sodium. It lathers beautifully, does not leave a ring around the tub, but, unfortunately, is not as healthy as the "hard" water.

High intakes of sodium are associated with hypertension in some people and increased calciuria (calcium in the urine). Sodium is the key dietary factor influencing urinary calcium loss.[3]

Oral Rehydration, Medical Missions, and a "White Powdery Substance."

The year was 1999 and I was going to Guatemala with a group of nursing, health, and language students from Liberty University to head up the medical/dental component of our missionary outreach. Dehydration due to heat and diarrheal illnesses is commonplace in Guatemala, so in an effort to be efficient before we left on the trip, I asked my students to prepare individual bags of powdered oral rehydration packets consisting of sugar, table salt, potassium chloride, and baking soda which, when mixed with water, would replenish water and electrolytes for those suffering from dehydration. See Table 5 for the recipe we used. To

PLAY YOUR HAND WELL

those in need, we would hand out the packets along with instructions on how to mix with water, how much water to use, when and how much to take, etc. Brilliant, I thought. If we make up these packets ahead of time, what a timesaver! What I hadn't anticipated was the reaction from customs officials at the airport to our suitcases containing bags of a white powdery substance!!! Having our rehydration packets confiscated at customs, we purchased the ingredients in Guatemala and made them up there. So much for efficiency!

Table 4. Recipe for Making Your Own Oral Rehydration Solution (ORS)

To 1 liter/quart of clean drinking water, add the following:

INGREDIENT	QUANTITY
Sugar	2 tablespoons
Table Salt	¼ teaspoon
Baking Soda	¼ teaspoon

- If you don't have any baking soda, add another 1/4 teaspoon of salt.

- If possible, add 1/2 cup orange juice or some mashed banana to improve the taste and provide some potassium.

- Drink sips of the ORS every five minutes until urination becomes normal. (It's normal to urinate four or five times a day.) Adults and large children should drink at least three quarts or liters of ORS a day until they are well.

- If you are vomiting, keep trying to drink the ORS. Your body will retain some of the fluids and salts you need even though you are vomiting. Remember to take only sips of liquids. Chilling the ORS may help.

- If you have diarrhea, keep drinking the ORS. The fluids will not increase the diarrhea.

CHAPTER 6
SOME VITAMINS SUPPLEMENTS CAN BE GOOD

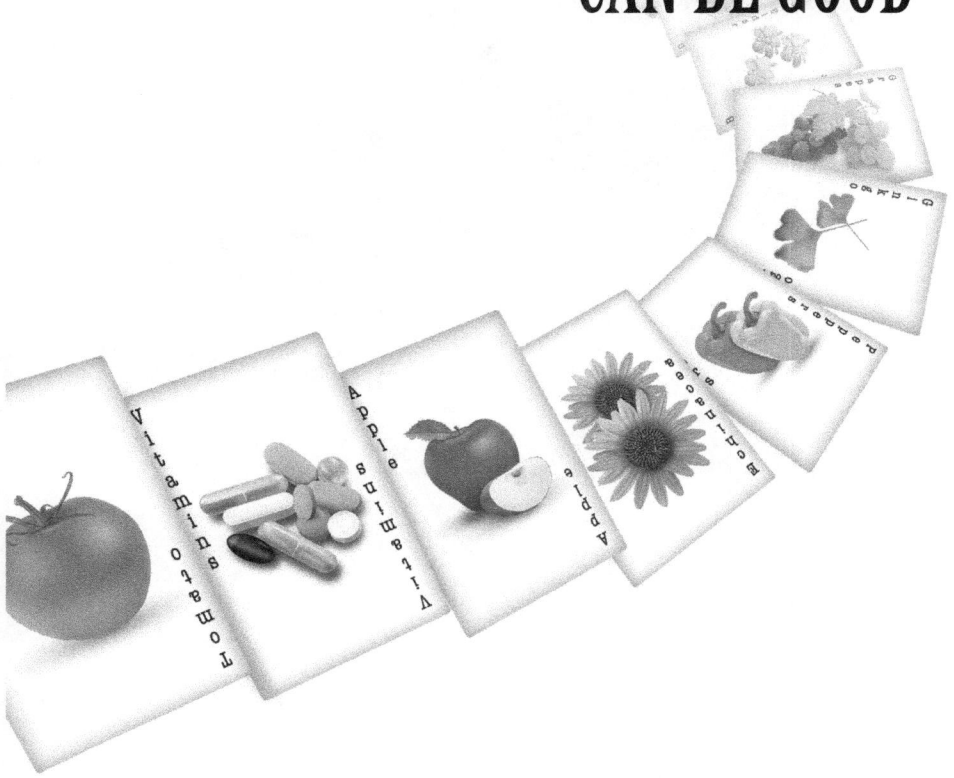

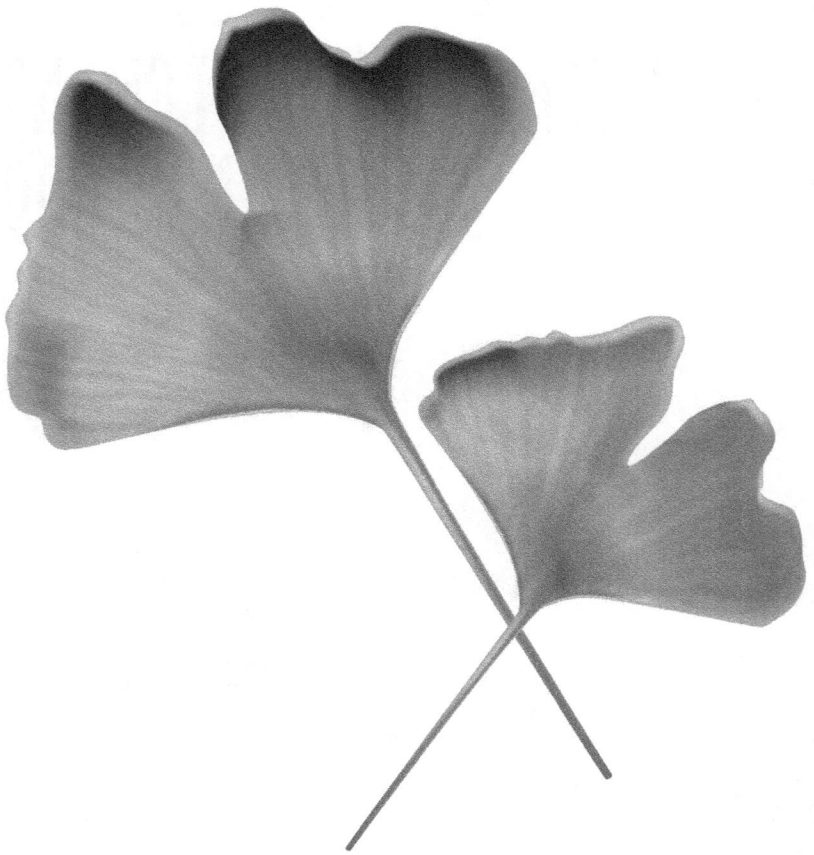

**Figure 5. Though the Best Source of Vitamins is Food;
Supplementation of Some Vitamins Can Be Beneficial.**

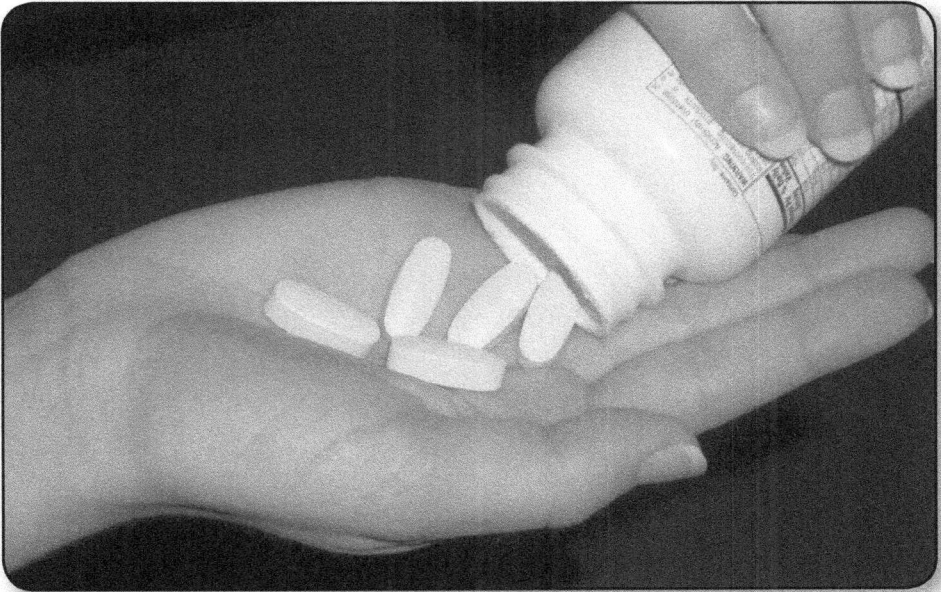

T he best source of vitamins is *food*, not pills. Fresh fruits and vegetables are teaming with beneficial nutrients, which provide more nourishment when consumed in combination with one another. Such nutrients demonstrate the *synergistic effect* meaning that the combined nutritional benefit is greater than the sum of the individual components. Because of this, the vitamins are actually more effective when eaten in food form, rather than isolated in supplement (pill) form. Many studies, particularly those with vitamin E and beta-carotene, which we will discuss later, support this.

In an ideal world, supplementation would perhaps not be necessary, but unfortunately, we do not live in an ideal world and vitamin supplementation can be beneficial.

> *Supplements should be used to support an already nutritious diet; not to compensate for a poor one.*

Antioxidants

Learning to play your hand well requires a thorough understanding of the category of vitamins and other plant-based compounds known as antioxidants. We have heard that *antioxidants* are good, but we may not be exactly sure what that means. If antioxidants are good things, then oxidants and oxidation must be bad, right? Pretty much. Think of *oxidation* as rust. Just like rust (oxidation) damages ferrous metal, oxidation in the body damages cells and tissue. The perpetrators of oxidation are destructive molecules known as free radicals, which are highly unstable, positively charged, oxygen-containing molecules that seek to combine with other molecules in the body in order to steal negatively charged electrons and achieve the neutrality that they desire. In so doing, they attack, damage, and destroy healthy cells and tissues. Free radicals are everywhere and are hard to get rid of. They are generated primarily from three sources:

- **Environmental** – includes air pollution, pesticides, herbicides, UV light and background radiation.
- **Internal** – from the body's own metabolism.
- **Stress factors** – aging, trauma, medications, disease, infection, psychological stress, and intense, strenuous physical exercise.[1]

Antioxidants act quite heroically and unselfishly in that they sacrifice themselves by donating electrons to the free radicals in order to spare the healthy cells and tissue. When they donate electrons, they, in effect, "die" but they die so that the cells of the body might live.

Don't Let Your LDL get Oxidized!

Remember earlier when we talked about LDL (bad) and HDL (good) cholesterol? We said that it wasn't so much the LDL level *per se* that contributed directly to heart disease, but rather the ease at which the LDL becomes oxidized. It attracts free radicals, oxidation occurs, and the *oxidized* LDL is viewed by the body as a foreign substance, and attacked by immune cells known as macrophages. It is this oxidized LDL that is the risk factor for heart disease, not just LDL by itself. If we can prevent this oxidation from occurring through the judicious use of antioxidants, then, even though the LDL levels may be higher than optimal, we can go a long way toward preventing heart disease. So, be sure to consume plenty of antioxidant vitamins on a daily basis and don't let your LDL get oxidized!

Where may antioxidants be found? Many plants contain *phytonutrients*, which are highly beneficial chemical compounds that demonstrate antioxidant activity. The body is another source and is able to manufacture its own antioxidants to some degree utilizing, among other things, minerals to be discussed later. Most antioxidants, however, have to be supplied on a regular basis by the diet. The three most important antioxidants are vitamin C, vitamin E, and beta-carotene.

Your Mother Knew: Vitamin C is Good for You!

She always made you drink extra orange juice when you started to come down with a cold and although it wasn't the magic bullet that you hoped it would be, it did seem to help. Vitamin C is a water-soluble antioxidant vitamin necessary for the hydroxylation of *proline*, an essential amino acid found in the connective tissue known as *collagen*. Collagen supports blood vessels and makes them strong and healthy so they don't leak. The vitamin C deficiency disease, known as scurvy, is characterized by bleeding, especially of the mouth and gums. Bleeding of the gums can be caused by other things as well, but in the absence of other factors, scurvy should be considered. Scurvy is not that common in the U.S., however, dentists are often the first to make the diagnosis; I may have seen it in my practice once or twice. Other symptoms of scurvy include fatigue and lethargy. British sailors were referred to as *"limeys"* because they were issued limes for their extended trips at sea to prevent the dreaded disease. The bleeding occurs due to lack of collagen, which causes the blood vessels to become weak, and, like old worn-out garden hoses, they leak. The symptoms of scurvy are characterized by the "4 Hs:"

- Hemorrhage
- Hyperkaratosis
- Hypochondriasis
- Hematologic abnormalities

Linus Pauling is the only person to have won two unshared Nobel Prizes, the Nobel Prize for Chemistry in 1954 for his research into the nature of the chemical bond, and the Nobel Peace Prize in 1962 for his efforts in the area of world peace and nuclear non-proliferation.[2] He is probably best known, however, for his landmark work entitled: *Vitamin C and the Common Cold* in which he maintained that the common cold can be controlled by proper nutrition and the use of vitamin C. He maintained that the RDA for vitamin C was too low (see Table 5) and would himself take doses well in excess of 2000 milligrams per day (sometimes as high as 10,000 mg/day!) As discussed earlier, I believe this to be way too much due to the potential to interfere with the role that folic acid and vitamin B_{12} play in lowering blood levels of homocysteine. The RDA has been set as the minimum level required to prevent a *deficiency*, but for *optimal* health, higher levels are probably required, especially for smokers. Cigarette smoke produces a large number of free radicals; therefore, more vitamin C is needed by smokers (better yet, just quit smoking!). My recommendation for most adults would be around 500 mg per day, with as much of that from *food* as possible. Some estimates are that it takes 900 mg from *supplements* to equal the antioxidant power of 60 mg vitamin C from *food!*[3] Avoid the chewable form of vitamin C which is highly acidic and can dissolve the enamel from your teeth! The best food sources of vitamin C are listed in Table 6.

> *Some estimates are that it takes 900 mg of vitamin C from supplements to equal the antioxidant power of 60 mg from food.*

Does vitamin C prevent the common cold? The research is inconclusive. An analysis of several studies with vitamin C showed an average reduction in the duration of colds by about 8% in adults and 14% in children; another study showed that vitamin C in doses of 250 mg to 1 g/day decreased the incidence of colds by 50% in a group of marathon runners, skiers and soldiers training in the Arctic.[4] Vitamin C may reduce the incidence and severity of colds by increasing production of the B and T cells which are an integral part of the immune system or possibly through antibacterial and antiviral properties. Some studies have found vitamin C to be ineffective in preventing colds. Other functions of vitamin C include:

- Vitamin C enhances iron absorption and is beneficial to take with iron supplements if indicated.

- Vitamin C plays an important role in the metabolism of norepinephrine, a neurotransmitter in the brain, which is important for regulating mood and energy levels, and explains why patients with scurvy exhibit lethargy and hypochondriasis.

- The First National Health and Nutrition Examination Study (NHANES I) found that the risk of death from cardiovascular diseases was 42% lower in men and 25% lower in women who consumed more than 50 mg/day of vitamin C and who regularly took vitamin C supplements, corresponding to a total vitamin C intake of about 300 mg/day.[5] The ability of vitamin C to prevent oxidation of LDL is the most likely explanation for this observation.

- Though the research is contradictory and inconclusive, some studies have shown vitamin C to be beneficial in the prevention of certain types of cancer, cataracts, stroke, and kidney stones.[6]

Table 5. Recommended Dietary Allowance (RDA) for Vitamin C*

LIFE STAGE	AGE	MALES (mg/day)	FEMALES (mg/day)
Children	1 – 3 years	15	15
Children	4 – 8 years	25	25
Children	9 – 13 years	45	45
Adolescents	14 – 18 years	75	65
Adults	19 years and older	90	75
Smokers	19 years and older	125	110
Pregnancy	18 years and younger	-	80
Pregnancy	19 years and older	-	85
Breastfeeding	18 years and younger	-	115
Breastfeeding	19 years and older	-	120

*As established by the Food and Nutrition Board of the Institute of Medicine, U.S. National Academy of Sciences.

PLAY YOUR HAND WELL

Table 6.   Food Sources of Vitamin C.

FOOD	SERVING	VITAMIN C (mg)
Orange Juice	¾ cup (6 ounces)	75
Grapefruit Juice	¾ cup (6 ounces)	60
Orange	1 medium	70
Grapefruit	½ medium	44
Strawberries	1 cup, whole	82
Tomato	1 medium	23
Sweet Red Pepper	½ cup, raw chopped	141
Broccoli	½ cup, cooked	58
Potato	1 medium, baked	26

Beta-Carotene in Foods is Good; in Supplement Form, Maybe Not!

Beta-carotene belongs to a colorful family of compounds known as *carotenoids*, which are found in yellow and dark green leafy fruits and vegetables such as carrots, squash, papaya, pumpkins, sweet potatoes, kale, spinach, and broccoli. Of the over 600 known carotenoids, there are six primary ones found in the diet: lycopene, beta-carotene, alpha-carotene, beta-cryptoxanthin, lutein, and zeaxanthin. Table 7 lists the primary carotenoids and their food sources.

Beta-Carotene is a precursor to vitamin A and is referred to as a provitamin because it is converted into active vitamin A as needed by the body. Active vitamin A is known as *retinol* and is necessary for healthy vision (remember your mother told you to eat your carrots and that you would see better because of it?), healthy skin (vitamin A is used in several acne medications), and for growth and immunity. It is found in liver, butter, and eggs. Unlike beta-carotene, active vitamin A is not an antioxidant and can be toxic when consumed in supplement form. Under the supervision of a health care professional, active vitamin A supplementation may be indicated for the management of symptoms related to the following:

- Xerophthalmia (dry eyes)

- Severe protein-energy malnutrition

- Measles (Remember Mary, on *Little House on the Prairie*? The popular book by Laura Ingalls Wilder mentioned that Mary contracted scarlet fever and became blind as a result. Blindness is not a typical complication of scarlet fever; therefore, it was most likely measles that caused Mary's blindness since measles depletes the body of active vitamin A).

- Tuberculosis

- HIV

- Retinitis Pigmentosa[7]

Like vitamin C, beta-carotene is a powerful antioxidant vitamin associated with many health benefits, especially in the area of reducing the risk of lung cancer and cardiovascular disease when taken in *food* form. In the early 1990s, there was strong evidence that the consumption of beta-carotene-rich fruits and vegetables decreased the risk of lung cancer. As a result, two large studies were undertaken to see if beta-carotene *supplements* would be as effective in decreasing lung cancer risk. The Alpha-Tocopherol Beta-Carotene Cancer Prevention Trial (ATBC) examined the lung cancer risk in Finnish male smokers and the Beta-Carotene and Retinol Efficacy Trial (CARET) looked at male and female smokers or asbestos-exposed workers. Those enrolled in the trials received beta-carotene supplements (20 mg daily in the ATBC; 30 mg daily in the CARET) or placebo. The research community was shocked when ATBC and CARET results found significant 18% and 28% *increases* in lung cancer risk, respectively, among those receiving the beta-carotene supplements.[8]

> *Beta-carotene from food decreased the risk of lung cancer; Beta-carotene from supplements made the cancer worse!*

Similarly, a significant 10% *increased* risk of cardiovascular death was associated with beta-carotene *supplementation* (15-50 mg), while beta-carotene consumption in the form of carotenoid-rich *foods* has shown a *decreased* risk of developing cardiovascular disease.[9] That's enough for me; I'm getting my beta-carotene from food, not pills! I do not recommend beta-carotene *supplementation*. Dr. Kenneth Cooper recommends a minimum of 15 mg of beta-carotene (15 mg beta-carotene equals 25,000 International Units) from *food* each day, which could be obtained from the following list of suggestions:

- ½ cup of cooked sweet potatoes, *or* 1 ½ medium carrots, *or* 2 mangoes
- ½ cup cooked pumpkin, *or* 1 ½ cups of cooked spinach
- ½ cup boiled spinach, 1 cup cantaloupe, *and* ½ raw carrot
- ½ cup boiled broccoli, 3 medium apricots, *and* ½ cup boiled carrots
- 1 medium papaya, ½ cup frozen spinach, *and* ½ baked sweet potato10

Another good source of beta-carotene is pumpkin seeds, so be sure to save your seeds from your pumpkin carving at Halloween time. Roast them, garnish with a light coating of olive oil, and you have one healthy and tasty snack!

Health benefits from the other carotenoids have been reported and have demonstrated promise in the management of macular degeneration, cataracts, and prostate cancer but more research is needed before specific recommendations can be made.[11]

Table 7. Food Sources of the Primary Carotenoids.

CAROTENOID	COLOR	FOOD SOURCES
Lycopene	Red	Tomatoes, watermelon, guava, pink grapefruit
Beta-carotene	Yellow-orange	Carrots, sweet potatoes, pumpkin, spinach, apricots
Alpha-carotene	Light yellow	Carrots, pumpkin
Beta-cryptoxanthin	Orange	Sweet red peppers, tangerines, papaya, persimmons
Lutein	Yellow	Kale, spinach, corn, collard greens, broccoli, eggs
Zeaxanthin	Yellow	Kale, spinach, corn, collard greens, broccoli, eggs

PLAY YOUR HAND WELL

Vitamin E

Figure 8. Vitamin E is One of the Most Powerful Antioxidants Known.

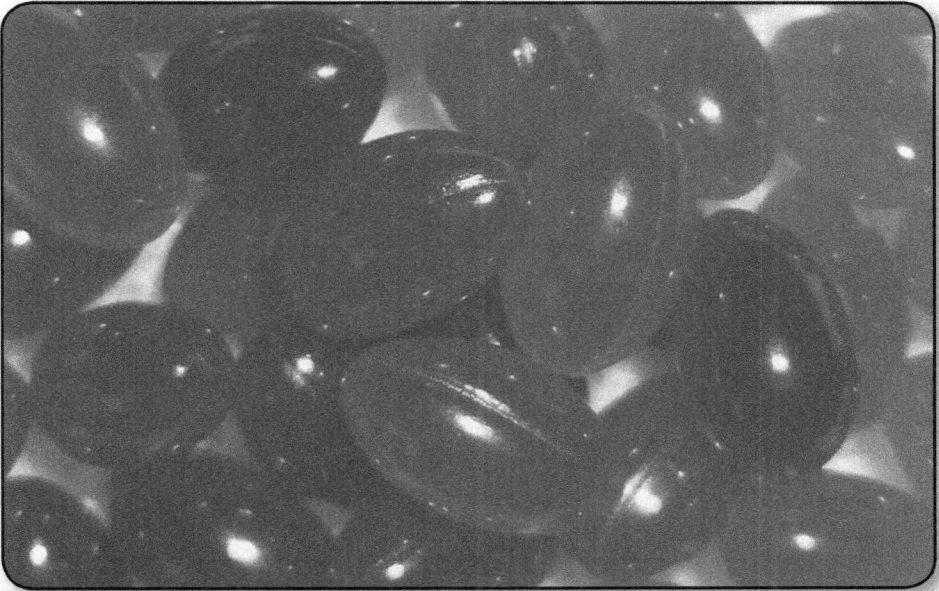

The chemical name for vitamin E is *tocopherol* which comes from two Greek words: *tokos* meaning "childbirth" and *pherein* meaning "to bear" since it was noted at its discovery in 1922 that this vitamin was necessary for pregnant rats to give birth.[12] Vitamin E is a powerful fat-soluble antioxidant which has been demonstrated to be effective in decreasing the risk of cardiovascular disease, largely through its ability to prevent the oxidation of LDL cholesterol. It also protects nerve cell membranes and is instrumental in the prevention of *hemolytic anemia* (the rupturing of red blood cells due to weakened membranes). Exciting new research has demonstrated *possible* reduction in the risks of amyotrophic lateral sclerosis (Lou Gehrig's Disease) and Alzheimer's disease.[13,14] Vitamin E works in concert with vitamin C to protect cells and membranes from oxidative damage caused by free radicals. It also demonstrates a "blood-thinning" effect, largely the result of its ability to limit platelet adhesion and by interfering with the action of vitamin K. Deficiency of vitamin E can result in neurologic disorders, hemolytic anemia, atherosclerosis, cataracts, and certain types of cancer. Over-supplementation with vitamin E can result in bleeding. Since vitamin E is a fat-soluble vitamin, it requires an intact and fully functioning digestive system for adequate absorption. Patients with celiac disease, cystic fibrosis, pancreatic, liver, gallbladder, and other diseases that would result in the inability to absorb vitamin E will demonstrate symptoms of vitamin E deficiency disorders.[15]

The richest dietary sources of vitamin E are wheat germ, nuts (especially almonds) and vegetable oils such as safflower and sunflower oil. Fruits and vegetables are generally not good sources of vitamin E.

Table 8 gives the RDA for vitamin E along with the safe upper limit (UL). Generally for adults, 200-800 mg per day from food and supplementation is recommended, however, as with vitamin C supplementation, vitamins in *food* form are more potent than in *pill* form as it may take up to 800 IU (1 International Unit of vitamin E = approximately 1 mg vitamin E) of vitamin E from *supplements* to equal the antioxidant potential of just 10 IU of vitamin E from *food!* [16]

> *It may take up to 800 IU of vitamin E from supplements to equal the antioxidant potential of just 10 IU of vitamin E from food.*

Oxidative damage increases with strenuous exercise, smoking, and aging, so higher daily doses are indicated in these situations; the upper limit should not be exceeded. Natural vitamin E (which may be labeled as d-alpha tocopherol, d-alpha-tocopherol, d-alpha tocopheryl acetate, or d-alpha-tocopheryl acetate) is preferred as it is better absorbed than the synthetic vitamin E. Synthetic vitamin E may be recognized by the insertion of the letter "l" after the "d" as in dl-alpha tocopherol, dl-alpha-tocopherol, dl-alpha tocopheryl acetate, or dl-alpha-tocopheryl acetate.[17]

Table 8. Recommended Dietary Allowance (RDA) and Safe Upper Limits (UL) for Vitamin E.*

LIFE STAGE	AGE	RDA (mg/day)	UL (mg/day)
Children	1 – 3 years	6	200
Children	4 – 8 years	7	300
Children	9 – 13 years	11	600
Adolescents	14 – 18 years	15	800
Adults	19 years and older	15	1000
Pregnancy	18 years and younger	15	808
Pregnancy	19 years and older	15	1000
Breastfeeding	18 years and younger	19	800
Breastfeeding	19 years and older	19	1000

*As established by the Food and Nutrition Board of the Institute of Medicine, U.S. National Academy of Sciences.

Your Mother Knew About Vitamin D, Too!

She might have been wrong in leading you to believe that if you ate your carrots you would have x-ray vision like Superman, but she was right about vitamin C and she was also right about vitamin D. Remember when she made you take your cod liver oil or encouraged you to play outside in the sunshine? She knew. Vitamin D is a hormone, really. A hormone is a chemical messenger produced by one organ of the body, which enters the bloodstream and has an effect on another organ of the body. Vitamin D is produced by the largest organ of the body, the skin, in response to sunlight. It enters the bloodstream and has an effect on the digestive tract by "telling" it to absorb calcium. Vitamin D is the sunshine vitamin and is necessary for calcium absorption. Without vitamin D, calcium is not absorbed; without calcium the bones are weak and diseases like rickets, in children, and osteomalacia, in adults are the result. Vitamin D deficiency is seen primarily in the following groups of people:

- Dark-skinned individuals. Since the pigment in the skin blocks some of the sun's rays necessary for vitamin D production (interestingly, O.J. Simpson was diagnosed with rickets as a child, but fortunately the diagnosis was made early enough for appropriate vitamin D therapy to preclude permanent skeletal problems; many are not so fortunate).

- The elderly. Lactose intolerance, which is fairly common in elderly persons, renders many unable to drink milk, a major source of vitamin D.

- Those who live in northern climates. Seasonal variations of sunlight reduce the skin's vitamin D production.

- Muslims. The clothing habits of some people block sunlight and reduce, if not eliminate, vitamin D production.[18]

The previous recommended intake for vitamin D of 200 IU/day for *infants, children and adolescents* has recently been increased to 400 IU/day as recommended by the American Academy of Pediatrics.[19] The Institute of Medicine of the U.S. National Academy of Sciences recommends the following levels of vitamin D for adults:

- Adults 19-50: 200 IU

- Adults 51-70: 400 IU

- Adults 71 and over: 600IU

- Pregnancy all ages: 200 IU

- Breastfeeding all ages: 200 IU

Because it is toxic in high doses, an upper limit of 2000 IU/day has been established by the U.S. Food and Nutrition Board of the Institute of Medicine.[20] Foods which provide the best sources of vitamin D include saltwater fish such as herring, salmon, and sardines and fish liver oil (cod liver oil). Eggs, veal, beef, and butter also provide some. In the U.S., milk is fortified with vitamin D and is a primary source for many individuals. Supplementation should be encouraged in those persons for whom deficiency is likely (see above).

The B Vitamins

I did my undergraduate work at Dickinson College in Carlisle, Pennsylvania, majoring in Biology. Students who conducted original research were provided with their own laboratories, complete with microscopes, lab supplies and instruments. Naturally, I wanted my own lab, so I decided to conduct original cancer research (what a motivating factor for the furthering of scientific knowledge!) My lab was a wonderful facility and was approximately 12' by 18.' I shared it with another Biology major (who was also my roommate) and we learned together. He learned about cancer research on mice from me and I learned about the presence of *Schistosomes* in turkey droppings from him! He kept a pair of orphaned screech owls in our lab and we would keep them well fed with mice left over from my research!

I was interested in a new "miracle cure" for cancer at the time known by several names including *"amygdalin," "laetrile,"* or *vitamin B$_{17}$*, a naturally occurring compound found in apricot seeds.[21] In the 1970s it was receiving considerable recognition for its anti-cancer activities and, since it was illegal to obtain in the U.S., many cancer patients were traveling to Mexico to receive treatment.

My inquisitive mind kicked in (along with the reward of obtaining my own research laboratory) and I decided to investigate the effectiveness of this compound on reducing the size of skin tumors in mice. My research took approximately six months and the results were presented in my senior thesis entitled: "The Effects of Amygdalin on the S91 Melanoma in ICR Mice."[22] I would find what other researchers before and since have concluded: Amygdalin does *not* work and it is not one of the B vitamins. Nevertheless, I learned invaluable expertise in conducting original research that year (1975), I had my own lab, and our pet screech owls were well-fed with mice!

Though there is no "vitamin B_{17}," there are eight other compounds that are truly B vitamins and I would like to take this opportunity to discuss their importance. The B vitamins act as *coenzymes* in the body, essentially assisting enzymes in various biochemical processes, including the production of energy in the form of ATP from glucose. One of the first signs of a deficiency of vitamin B is that you feel tired and run-down from this inability to fully-generate ATP from glucose. The B vitamins are water-soluble and they need to be replenished on a regular basis. With the exception of niacin, which is toxic to the liver in large doses, and vitamin B_6, which can cause nerve damage when taken in large doses, appropriate supplementation with the B vitamins is often recommended as an adjunct to a healthy, well-balanced diet.

Vitamin B_1 (thiamin) is necessary for the production of energy from glucose and also for the synthesis of another neurotransmitter, acetylcholine, which is necessary for proper nerve function. The vitamin B_1 deficiency disease is known as *beriberi* and is seen in countries where "polished" rice is the main staple. Polished rice results in the removal of the bran layer of the rice and renders the grain devoid of thiamin. Alcohol destroys thiamin, and a neuro-degenerative disorder known as *Wernicke-Korsakoff syndrome* is seen with chronic alcohol abuse. The best food sources of thiamin include whole grains, nuts, seeds, and legumes.

Vitamin B$_2$ (riboflavin) is also involved with energy production. Milk is a good source of riboflavin as are whole grains and leafy green vegetables. Since it is destroyed by light, it is advised that milk be purchased in containers of cardboard or opaque plastic to prevent the passage of light. A deficiency of riboflavin results in *angular cheilosis* (cracked, bleeding fissures at the corners of the mouth) and *glossitis* (inflammation of the tongue). I returned from a mission trip to Guatemala with angular cheilosis from not consuming green leafy vegetables, whole grains, or milk for a period of three weeks (I had given all my vitamin B supplements to the local villagers who needed them more than I did).

Vitamin B$_3$ (niacin) functions in energy production along with the previous two. It also is capable of lowering LDL (bad) cholesterol and elevating the HDL (good) cholesterol when taken in megadoses (3 grams per day). One must be extremely careful of using niacin in large doses, however, due to the toxic effect on the liver. Niacin should be used for this purpose only under the careful supervision of a physician or other health-care professional and the liver enzymes (ALT and AST) should be monitored by blood tests every six weeks to check for liver complications. The tolerable upper limit (UL) has been set at 35 mg/day for adults. Good sources of niacin include legumes, mushrooms, wheat bran, and peanuts. The niacin deficiency disease is known as *pellagra* and, in contrast to the "4 Hs" of scurvy, is characterized by the "4 Ds:"

- Dermatitis
- Diarrhea
- Dementia
- Death

Biotin is also a coenzyme. Its best food sources include liver and egg yolks; a deficiency of this vitamin causes nausea, dermatitis, and hair loss. Rarely is a biotin deficiency the cause of hair loss; shampoos often attempt to capitalize on this, but there is no evidence that taking biotin supplements or incorporating it into shampoo will reverse hair loss or thinning hair.

Pantothenic acid is involved with energy production along with the other B vitamins. A deficiency is rare since it is found in a great variety of foods (hence the name *"pan,"* Greek for *every* or *all*). Food sources include meat, whole grains and legumes.

Vitamin B$_6$ (pyridoxine) is necessary for protein metabolism. Since antibodies, hemoglobin, and the neurotransmitters *serotonin* and *dopamine*, are all proteins, a deficiency of vitamin B$_6$ would result in a depressed immune system, anemia, and depression (due to the underproduction of serotonin and dopamine). Exciting research has demonstrated a therapeutic effect for vitamin B$_6$ in the management of carpal tunnel syndrome, pre-menstrual syndrome, and clinical depression. Nerve damage occurs in doses approaching 1000 mg/day; the safe upper limit for adults has been established at 100 mg/day. Whole grains, meat, leafy greens, and legumes are good sources of vitamin B$_6$.

Folic acid is required for the synthesis of RNA and DNA (needed for cell division). Deficiency results in elevated levels of homocysteine (discussed earlier), neural tube defects such as *spina bifida*, and a type of anemia known as *megaloblastic anemia* (red blood cells unable to divide, grow bigger and bigger and become ineffective in transporting oxygen). Folic acid status is critical, particularly during pregnancy to prevent neural tube defects. Good sources of folic acid are raw fruits and vegetables such as broccoli and legumes.

Vitamin B$_{12}$ (cobalamin) works in conjunction with folic acid in the synthesis of RNA and DNA and in lowering levels of homocysteine. A deficiency of vitamin B$_{12}$ causes nerve damage and megaloblastic or pernicious anemia, and may contribute to *elevated* levels of homocysteine (hyperhomocysteinemia), and poor cognition.[23] Since the best sources of vitamin B$_{12}$ are meats and animal products, deficiency symptoms are likely to appear in vegans (strict vegetarians) who fail to supplement accordingly. Table 9 summarizes the adult RDA, function, deficiency and toxicity symptoms, and food sources for all the B vitamins.

: **L**earning to play your hand well
: **L** requires a thorough understanding of the category of vitamins
and other plant-based compounds
known as *antioxidants.*

Table 9. Recommended Adult Dietary Allowance (RDA), Function, Deficiency and Toxicity Symptoms, and Food Sources for the B Vitamins.

VITAMIN	RDA* (mg/day) MALE	RDA* (mg/day) FEMALE	FUNCTION
Thiamin	1.2	1.1	coenzyme; energy production
Riboflavin	1.3	1.1	coenzyme; energy production
Niacin	16	14	energy production; lowers cholesterol
Biotin	30**	30**	coenzyme
Pantothenic Acid	5	5	energy production; wound healing
Vitamin B$_6$	1.3 (1.7 if > 50)	1.3 (1.5 if > 50)	protein metabolism
Folic Acid	400**	400** (600 during preg.)	necessary for cell division (production of RNA and DNA)
Vitamin B$_{12}$	2.4**	2.4**	assists folic acid in the production of RNA and DNA

DEFICIENCY	TOXICITY	FOOD SOURCES
beriberi; Wernicke-Korsakoff	none	whole grains, nuts, seeds, legumes
angular cheilosis; glossitis	none	milk, whole grains, leafy greens
pellagra	flushing, itching, jaundice, hepatitis	wheat bran legumes, chicken, salmon, tuna, peanuts
nausea, dermatitis, hair loss	none	liver, egg yolks
delayed growth; dermatitis	none; mild diarrhea with doses > 10 g/day	meat, whole grains, legumes
depressed immune system; anemia, depression	nerve damage in doses > 1000 mg/ day	whole grains, meat, leafy greens, legumes
elevated levels of homocysteine; spina bifida; megalobastic anemia	none	raw fruits and vegetables, broccoli, legumes
pernicious anemia; elevated levels of homocysteine; impaired cognition?	none	animal products; meat

CHAPTER 7

SOME MINERAL SUPPLEMENTS ARE GOOD, TOO!

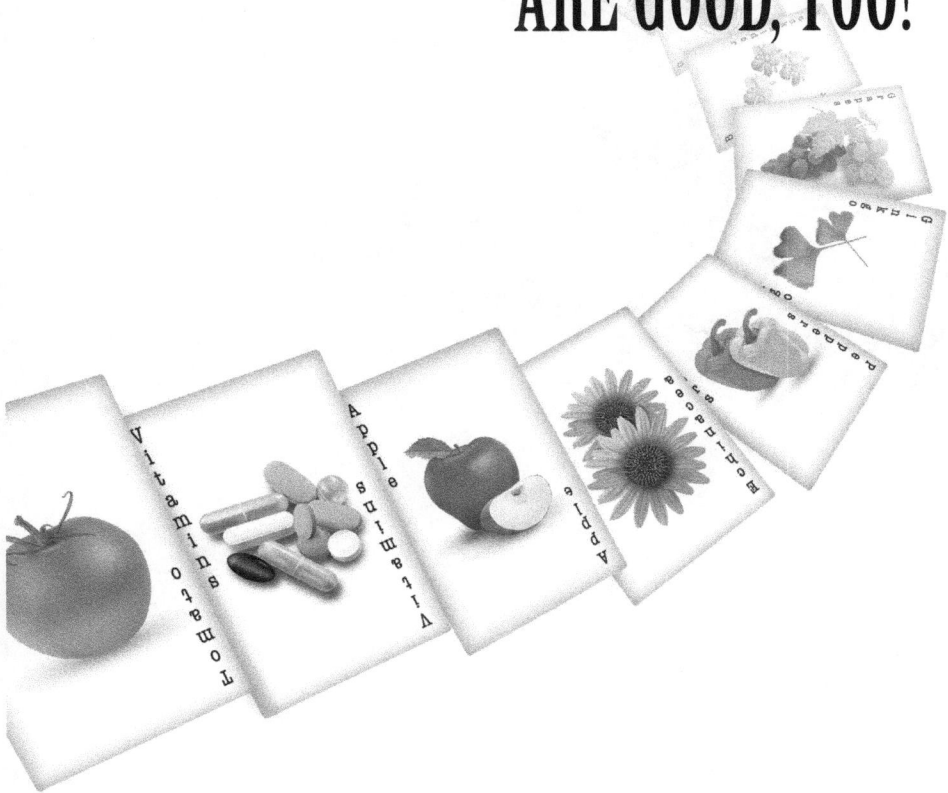

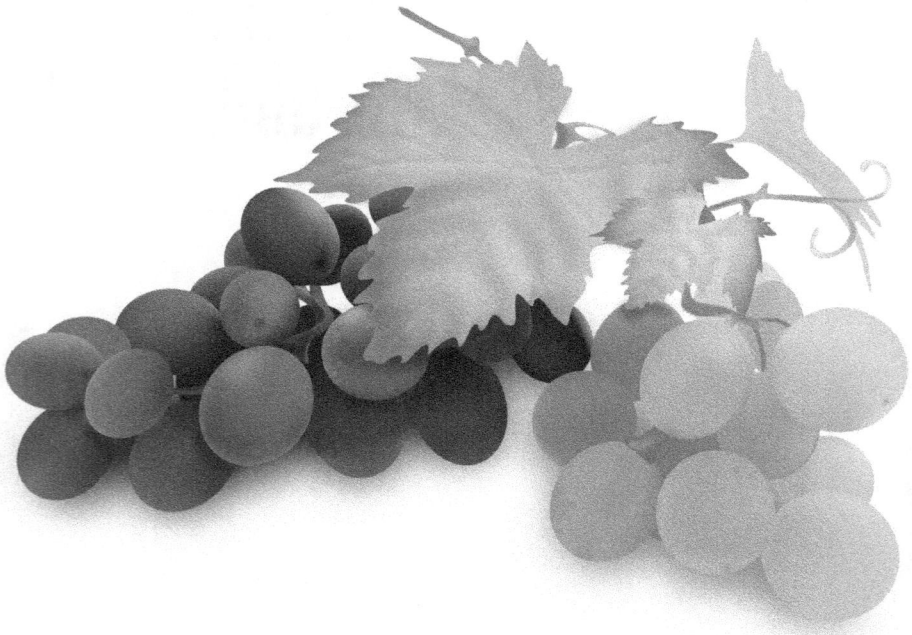

Minerals are elements that originate in the earth and cannot be made by living organisms. Plants obtain minerals from the soil, and most of the minerals in our diets come directly from plant, or indirectly from animal sources. Minerals may also be present in the water we drink. There are at least 24 different minerals that are essential to maintaining good health. Some we know a great deal about; others very little. Let's look at a few of the more important ones.

Calcium is Good; Fish is Good; Eat Sardines and Get Both!

Calcium may be thought of as a "wonder mineral" because it contributes to health in so many ways, some of which we are just beginning to appreciate. Most Americans get their calcium from dairy products, most Asians get theirs from dark-green leafy vegetables and tofu, and still others, particularly those with lactose intolerance, may get their calcium from supplements. Regardless of where one gets his/her calcium, the health benefits of this mineral are enormous! Let's begin with the obvious: calcium is needed to produce strong, healthy bones.

> *Calcium is the currency, the bones are the bank, and the bank is going to close around age 30!*

Calcium is the currency, the bones are the bank, and the bank is going to close around age 30. It is extremely important, therefore, for children and adolescents to obtain adequate intake of calcium during the bone forming years before the "bank" closes. Though most studies indicate that bone is *built* from 0-30 years of age resulting in peak bone mass at around age 30, *maintained* from 30-40, and *lost* from 40 on, some suggest that peak bone mass may actually occur much earlier.[1,2] The child needs to ensure that he/she has received adequate intake of calcium (and Vitamin D) and continues throughout the lifespan to cover for the losses which are inevitable later in life and which may lead to osteoporosis. The primary strategies for reducing the risk of osteoporosis are to maximize development of peak bone mass during growth and to reduce, through diet and weight-bearing exercise, bone loss later in life. Maximizing peak bone density protects against fracture at any age. Children who avoid milk have a bone fracture rate 1.75 times higher than expected compared to children who drink milk.[3] An upward trend in calcium requirements has occurred in Europe and North America in the last 15 years. The Food and Nutrition Board of the Institute of Medicine published its Adequate Intakes (AIs) for calcium data in 1997 and is presented in Table 10.

Table 10. Adequate Intakes (AI) for Calcium by Age for the United States and Canada.[4]

AGE	AI (mg/day)
0-6 months	210
6-12 months	270
1-3 years	500
4-8 years	800
9-18 years	1300
19-50 years	1000
51 and over	1200
Pregnant women (< 19)	1300
Pregnant women (> 19)	1000
Lactating women (< 19)	1300
Lactating women (> 19)	1000

We think of calcium as locked inside the bones in a static situation, when in reality it is constantly moving back and forth between the bones and the blood where it maintains a relatively constant blood level and participates in a host of bodily functions:

- Calcium is as important as fiber in helping to reduce the risk of colon cancer.[5,6] The mechanism by which calcium reduces the risk of colon cancer is thought to be related to its ability to bind with bile and free fatty acids, thereby reducing irritation to the lining of the colon.[7]

- Dietary calcium reduces the risk of high blood pressure and ischemic stroke; calcium deficiency is likely the main cause of the pregnancy-induced hypertension condition known as *preeclampsia*.[8,9]

- Calcium reduces the risk of kidney stones.[10] Years ago, it was thought that kidney stones were the result of *too much* calcium in the diet. One plausible explanation for how dietary calcium reduces the risk of kidney stones, is that when the body is deficient in calcium, it overcompensates by pulling it from the bones which results in elevated blood calcium and subsequent calcium precipitation in the kidney.

- Calcium has been shown to help alleviate symptoms associated with PMS.[11]

Vitamin D is necessary to ensure adequate calcium absorption. Because vitamin D is made by the skin in response to sunlight, for those individuals who cannot obtain exposure to the sun, vitamin D supplementation is recommended (see RDA guidelines in the previous chapter. Since vitamin D is toxic, the tolerable upper limit of 2000 IU/day should not be exceeded.

As we have already seen, fish is good. It is a good source of protein and omega-3 fat. Since our Mediterranean, Eskimo, and Asian friends consume much more fish than we Americans, heart disease among these populations is rare.[12] Combine fish and its heart-healthy properties with calcium and you have a winning combination. Many individuals from the Mediterranean area and in Asian cultures consume sardines and other fish, and various soups made from the bones of the fish. Calcium is obtained by eating sardines, bones and all, and in the case of soup, the calcium from the fish bones leaches into the nutrient-rich broth. Finally, tofu, made from the soybean, is an excellent source of calcium *and* high quality protein.

Figure 9. Sardines Are a Great Source of Calcium, As Well As Protein and the Good, Omega-3 Fats.

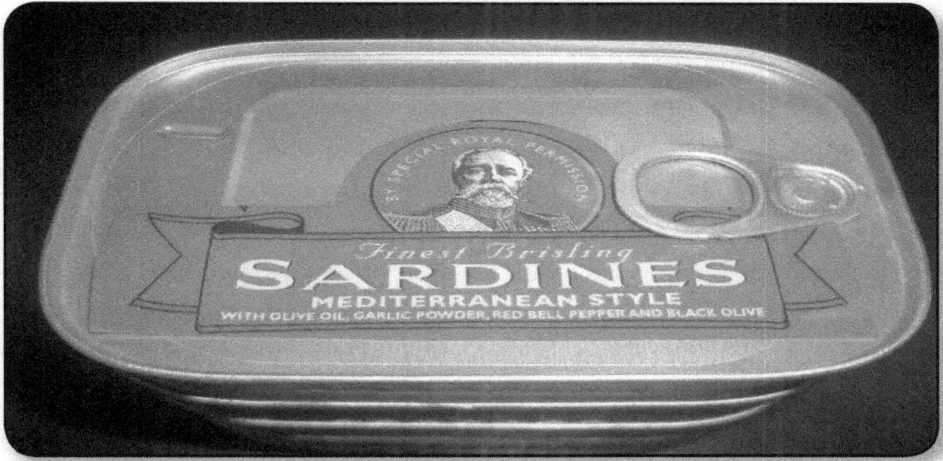

Other Minerals

Magnesium is necessary for healthy nerves, bone, and muscle. It is necessary for the proper functioning of the heart muscle, especially for muscle *relaxation* when the heart is at rest between beats. Magnesium is often given during heart surgery to prevent arrhythmia (irregular heart beat). Because it increases the osmolarity of the intestine causing an influx of water, it promotes peristalsis and is frequently used as a laxative. Magnesium also plays a role in improving glucose tolerance and in reducing the incidence of kidney stone formation. A constituent of the green plant pigment chlorophyll, it is found in leafy greens. Nuts, seafood, and whole grains are also good sources of magnesium.

    Iron is an important mineral, which is necessary for the production of the oxygen-carrying protein found in our red blood cells known as *hemoglobin*. Dietary iron comes from both plant and animal sources. Excess iron is stored in the liver, spleen, and bone marrow and eliminated primarily through blood loss. Iron supplementation may be indicated for children, some endurance athletes, especially females, in pregnancy, and in cases of malnutrition and disease states such as iron-deficiency anemia. For sedentary middle-aged men and those with too much iron (iron overload) iron supplementation is *not* indicated. Because it is easily oxidized, some have suggested an association between excessive iron intake and heart disease; a single dose of 180 mg may be lethal.[13] *Phytates* (phosphorous containing compounds found in whole grains, bran, and soy products), *tannins* (compounds found in tea) and calcium *decrease* the absorption of iron; iron supplements should not be taken with milk. Vitamin C, on the other hand *increases* the absorption of iron. Too much iron is toxic to the liver and interferes with the absorption of copper and zinc. Iron deficiency disease (iron deficiency anemia) remains a major nutritional disease in many parts of the world and is seen most often in women of childbearing age, children, adolescents, and athletes.

Copper is also required by the body in order to produce the antioxidant enzyme, *superoxide dismutase* (SOD) and is necessary for the transport of iron, for the production of the connective tissue collagen, and for muscle and nerve function. Some have suggested that *aneurisms* (ballooning of the wall of the artery due to insufficient collagen production) may be due, in part, to a deficiency in copper. A copper deficiency can be caused by too much zinc and results in elevated cholesterol and anemia; anemia results from:

- Decreased transport of iron.
- Increased destruction of red blood cells due to decreased levels of SOD.
- Blood loss due to weakened blood vessels caused by decreased collagen production.

Zinc is necessary for the body to produce the antioxidant enzyme, *superoxide dismutase* (SOD) which plays a major role in protecting red blood cells from oxidation caused by free oxygen radicals. Zinc also plays a role in growth and immunity. Phytates and iron both decrease the absorption of zinc, which is found in animal products, meat, seafood, and whole grains. Too much zinc, from over supplementation, can result in depletion of copper, nausea, vomiting, impaired immune function, and a lowered level of HDL.

Selenium is necessary for the production of yet another antioxidant enzyme, *Glutathione peroxidase* (GPO). Selenium also assists vitamin E and may be useful in preventing prostate cancer. A deficiency of selenium produces a progressive cardiomyopathy known as *Keshan disease*. Loss of hair and nails may result from over supplementation with selenium; a safe upper limit of 400 mcg/day has been established. Food sources of selenium include Brazil nuts, organ meats, and grains.

Sodium is the main positively charged ion (atom with a charge) found *outside* the cells of the body. Water is attracted to sodium and diets high in sodium promote and increase the fluid volume resulting in an increase in blood pressure. Sodium chloride (table salt) is the main source of sodium in the diet and western diets are typically very high in salt (sodium). Salt is an excellent preservative and is used in canned and processed foods in large amounts to prevent bacterial growth; a deficiency of sodium is rare, but can occur since sodium is lost through the urine, and in sweating, diarrhea, and vomiting; muscle cramps may result when sodium levels get too low. The Food and Nutrition Board of the Institute of Medicine has established the following adequate intake levels (AI) for *sodium* and for *salt (sodium chloride)*:

AGE	SODIUM (mg/day)	SALT (mg/day)
19-50 years	1500	3800
51-70 years	1300	3300
71 and over	1200	3000

Potassium is the main positively charged ion found *inside* the cells of the body. A deficiency of potassium is much more common than a sodium deficiency and is often caused by *diuretics* (high blood pressure medications), and dehydration from vomiting, sweating and diarrhea. Muscle cramps, confusion, and irregular heartbeats can occur (too much potassium from over supplementation can also cause irregular heartbeats). Potassium is found in raw fresh fruits and vegetables and unlike sodium, which often causes your blood pressure to go up, potassium from fresh fruits and vegetables makes your blood pressure go down. Bananas, raisins, orange juice, baked potatoes with skin, and tomato juice are excellent sources. The Food and Nutrition Board of the Institute of Medicine has established 4700 mg/day as the adequate intake level (AI) of potassium for adults over 19.

With the exception of calcium, iron, for those at risk groups mentioned above, and possibly magnesium, mineral supplementation, unless directed by a physician or other health care provider is probably not a good idea for the average adult. As we have seen, these minerals are involved in many complex biochemical processes throughout the body and there are many interactions and toxicity symptoms, which occur when large doses are taken in supplement form. Minerals often compete with one another in the body and supplementation can drive complex chemical reactions one way or another throwing the whole system out of balance. Vitamin and mineral overdosing is not a problem when vitamins and minerals are taken in food form.

Regardless of where one gets his/
her calcium, the health benefits
of this mineral are enormous!

Table 11. Recommended Adult Dietary Allowance (RDA), Function, Deficiency and Toxicity Symptoms, and Food Sources for the Several Important Minerals.

MINERAL	RDA* (mg/day) MALE	RDA* (mg/day) FEMALE	FUNCTION
Calcium***	1000; 1200 if >50	1000; 1200 if >50	muscle and bone health; lowers risks of high blood pressure, colon cancer, and PMS
Magnesium	420	320	nerve, muscle, and bone health; improves glucose tolerance, reduces risk of kidney stones
Iron	8	18 (27 during preg.)	manufacture of hemoglobin
Copper	900**	900**	SOD, iron transport, collagen, muscle and nerve
Zinc	11	8	SOD, growth, immunity
Selenium	55**	55**	GPO, assists vitamin E, may prevent prostate cancer

*   As established by the Food and Nutrition Board of the Institute of Medicine, U.S. National Academy of Sciences.
** Micrograms/day. 1 mcg = microgram = 1/1000th of a milligram = 1/100,000th of a gram.
*** RDA for calcium has not been established; Adequate Intakes (AI) are given instead.

DEFICIENCY	TOXICITY	FOOD SOURCES
high blood pressure; kidney stones; osteoporosis	interferes with the absorption of other minerals like iron and fluoride	milk, sardines, tofu, dark green leafy vegetables, calcium supplements
irregular heart beat (arrhythmias); atherosclerosis	diarrhea	greens such as spinach and Swiss chard, almonds, brown rice, oat bran; "hard" water
anemia	liver disease; heart disease?	red meat; leafy greens (kale and spinach)
anemia, aneurisms?, elevated cholesterol	vomiting	liver, shellfish, cashews, almonds, sunflower seeds, hazelnuts, and whole grains
delayed growth	nausea, vomiting; decreases immune function, HDL and copper	oysters, crab, beef, turkey (dark meat), whole grains
Keshan disease (heart disease)	Loss of hair and nails – seen in a region in China	brazil nuts, seafood, pork, brown rice, whole grains

CHAPTER 8

HERBAL MEDICINALS:
THE GOOD, THE BAD, AND THE "WE DON'T REALLY KNOW"

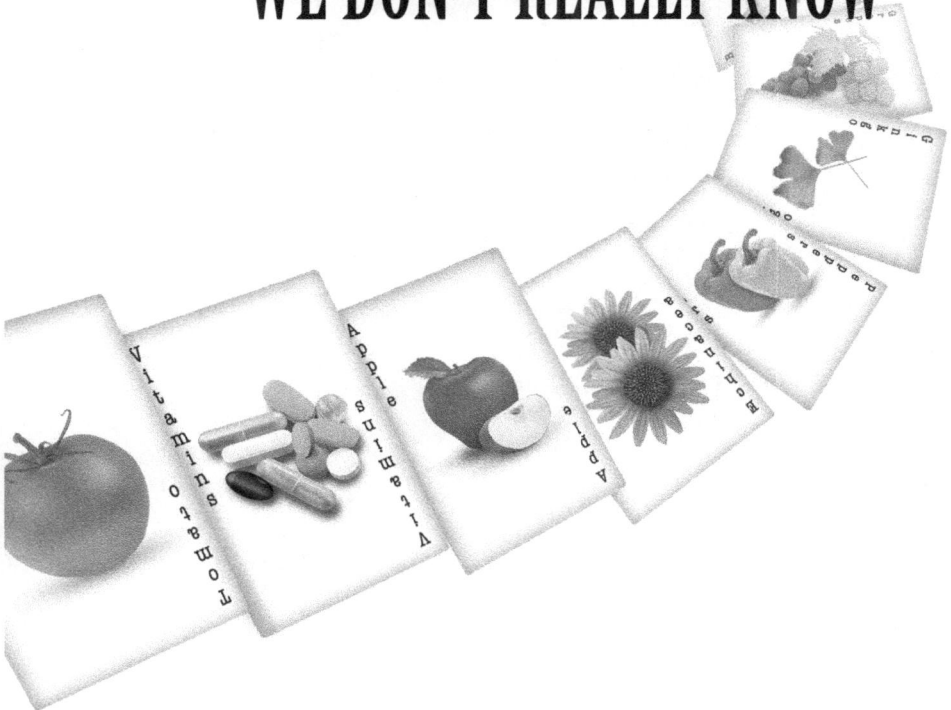

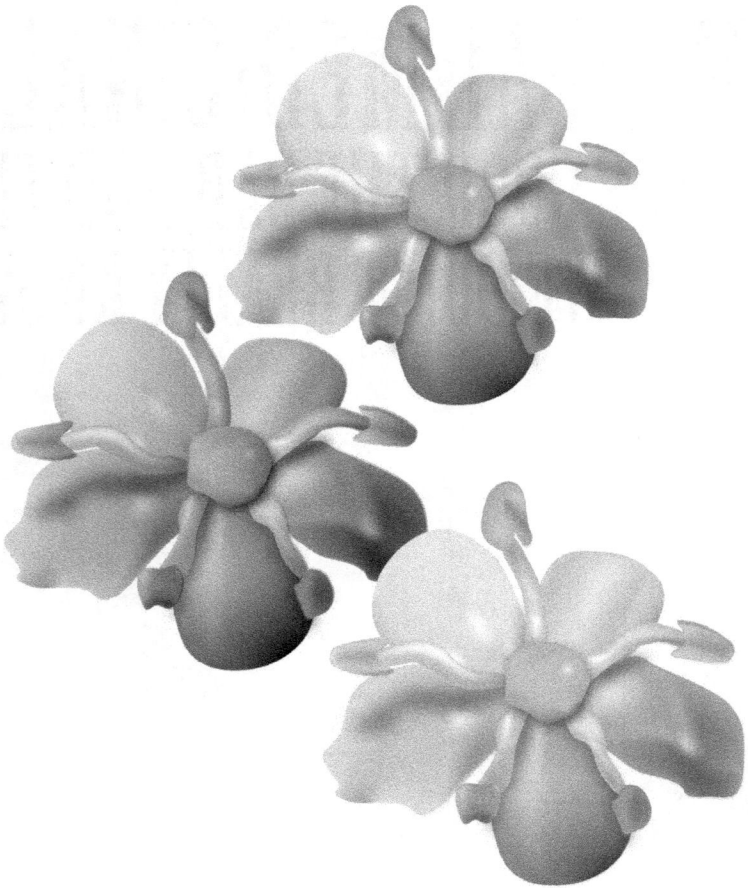

Man has recognized the medicinal properties of herbs for millennia. Historically, herbs have been used to numb our pain, to calm our fears, to give us energy, to help us sleep, to treat our infections and to heal our wounds. Our first commercially available pharmaceutical preparations came from herbal products and even today many of our synthetic modern medicines are derived from plant-based compounds. Relatively speaking, the U.S. has been late to appreciate the value of herbal medicines, which have always been held in high esteem in oriental countries and Europe. But that is beginning to change as many U.S. consumers and scientists alike have come to recognize the tremendous therapeutic benefits that many herbs have to offer.

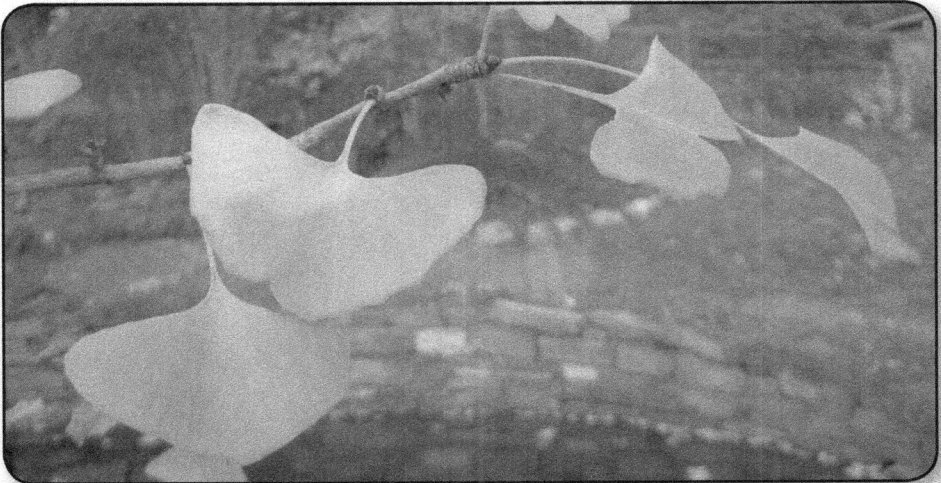

Ginkgo
(Ginkgo biloba)

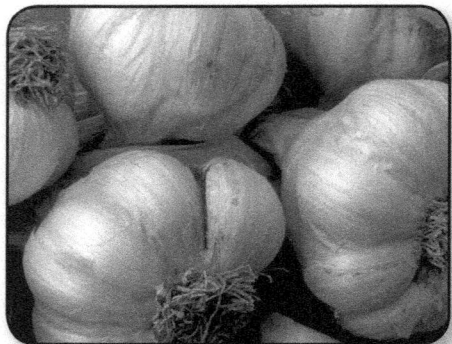

Garlic
(Allium sativum)

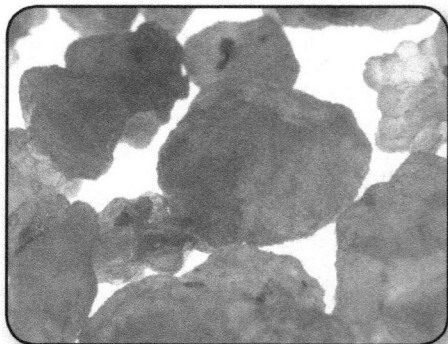

Myrrh
(Commiphora myrrha)

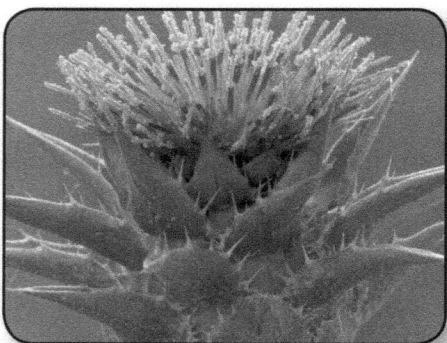

Milk Thistle
(Silybum arianum)

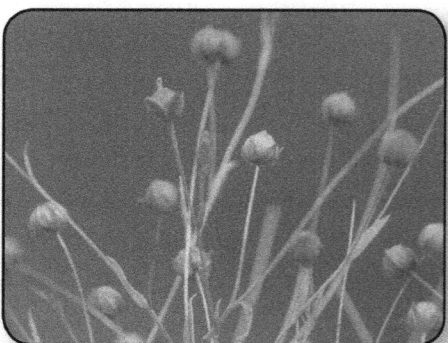

Flax
(Linum usitatissimum)

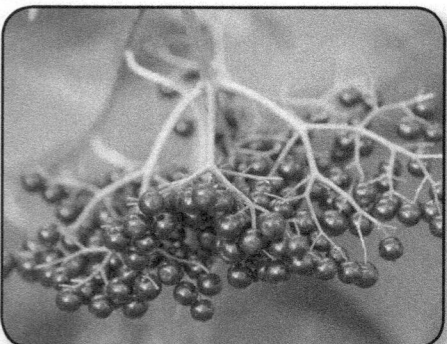

Black Elder
(Sambucus nigra)

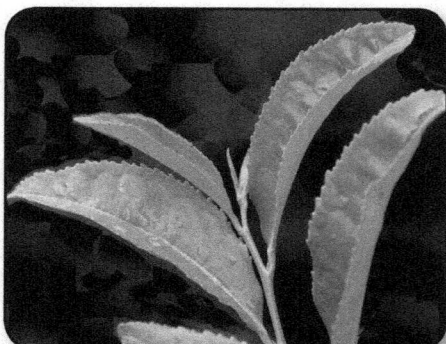

Green Tea
(Camellia sinensis)

PLAY YOUR HAND WELL

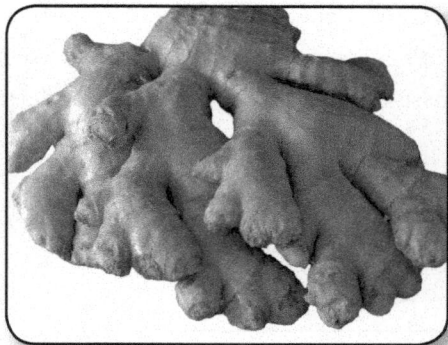

Ginger
(Zingiber officinale)

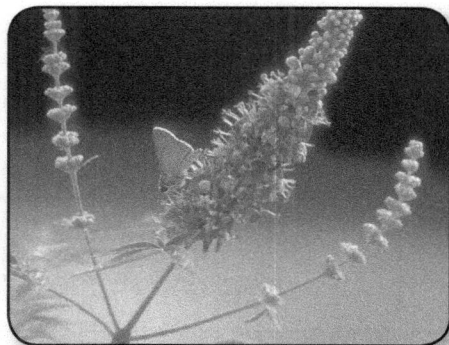

Chaste Tree
(Vitex agnus-castus)

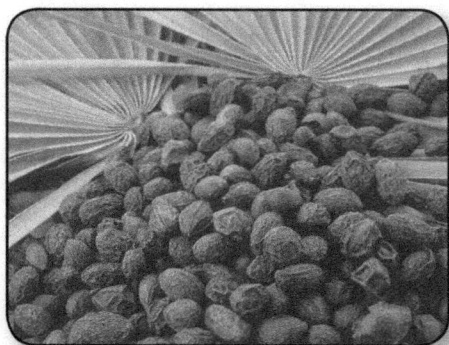

Saw Palmetto
(Serenoa repens)

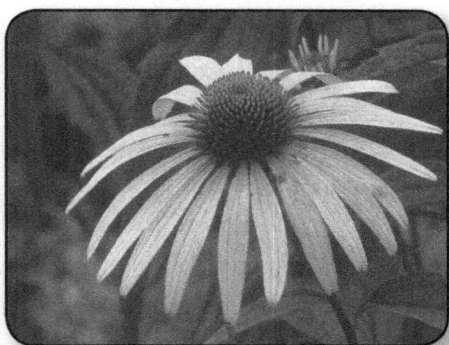

Echinacea
(Echinacea species)

As with vitamins, many herbal compounds demonstrate the *synergistic effect* in that their combined therapeutic value is greater than the sum of the individual components. To put it another way, the herbal compounds are usually more effective when taken together as they exist in nature (i.e. in the herb or plant) rather than isolated from the plant and put into the form of a supplement or pill (the music produced by a symphony is more wonderful and of a greater dimension than the music from each individual instrument). In addition to the synergistic effect, many herbs provide preventive benefits in assisting to keep us healthy so that we don't have to be treated when we are sick. Finally, when used properly, herbs are much less toxic and possess fewer side effects than modern pharmaceutical preparations.

> *Herbs are gifts from God; they heal the body, restore the mind, and stir the soul.*

Many, such as *Ephedra* can cause elevated blood pressures to the point that heart attack and stroke have been reported. Others, though they provide beneficial properties, can be toxic to the liver and interact with other known herbs and traditional medicines so that they should not be used without proper medical supervision. The following herbs were chosen on the basis of their therapeutic value from clinical trials and their record of safety. There are many more I could have included, but neither space nor time would permit. Though we have recently come to learn much about the medicinal qualities of herbal preparations, still, there's a lot we really don't know about them. Pharmaceutical companies just don't like to research anything that can't be patented, and herbal products rarely have patents. There are some exceptions: *Ginkgo biloba* is one of those exceptions. A few different patents have been awarded for a concentrated extract of Ginkgo; one such extract is EGb-761® which was developed by Schwabe Pharmaceuticals of Karlsruhe, Germany. EGb-761® works. I know; I did the research and this is my story:

My *Ginkgo biloba* Story

In 1998 I was teaching the human nutrition course at Liberty University. A student approached me one day after class and said: "I have been reading about an herb named *Ginkgo biloba* and that it can improve memory. Does it really work?" After some hesitation, my reply was: "I don't know, but I'll get back to you." The student was not satisfied with the answer, but politely smiled and slowly walked away to attend another class. I returned to my office; his question lingered. I did a brief search of the literature and learned very little. There had been some research with Ginkgo, mainly in Europe, but very little in the U.S. As I would learn later, this is often the case with botanical herb research since they are not protected by patents; there is little incentive for pharmaceutical companies to conduct clinical efficacy trials. Several weeks passed. The student returned once more with a rephrased question: "Dr. Mix, what have you learned about *Ginkgo biloba*, does it work or not?" "I don't know any more than the last time you asked me," I replied, "but we're going to find out." Thus began what would become, to my knowledge, the largest clinical trial ever conducted on the effects of *Ginkgo biloba* on cognitively-intact (healthy) seniors.[1]

It would be four years before I could give him his answer, however, and there would be such an incredible amount of work to do that my head would spin. We would need:

- An expert psychologist or neuropsychologist who was familiar with administering various cognitive assessment measures (memory tests).

- Enough people who would be willing to participate in such a study using a *double-blind* format. The term double blind means that neither the investigator nor the participant knows whether or not he is receiving the actual treatment (in this case, Ginkgo), or a placebo (sugar pill with no therapeutic value).

- Permission from the IRB (Institutional Review Board) of Liberty University to conduct such a trial.

- Students who would be willing to help with scheduling, making phone calls, recruiting, administering memory tests, etc.

- Money.

We were able to obtain all but the last one. In order to attract potential sources of funding, you need to demonstrate that you know how to appropriately conduct a clinical trial; in short, you need a track record, and you need to have a product, which at least has the potential to work. We had neither. Fortunately, I was able to locate a very talented neuropsychologist familiar with clinical research and cognitive assessment who was willing to assist me. But we desperately needed money so I applied the Willie Sutton philosophy (Willie Sutton was the famous bank robber who, when asked why he robbed banks replied: "'cause that's where the money is"). Who's got the money for research? Why, pharmaceutical companies, of course, so that's where I would concentrate my efforts. I searched for companies that made and sold Ginkgo products and my search lead me to one of the largest manufacturers of Ginkgo biloba supplements, Dr. Willmar Schwabe Pharmaceutical Company of Karlsruhe, Germany. The people at Schwabe were most intrigued with our efforts to conduct research on their product and their curiosity was sufficiently piqued to the point that they invited us to visit their facilities in Germany! Hoping, that we could convince them to fund us, we excitedly accepted their offer; if nothing else, at least we would have a free trip to Germany!

We flew to Frankfurt, Germany and proceeded to take the train to Karlsruhe. The German countryside was beautiful and reminded me of my former hometown in Pennsylvania. I spoke enough German to get by and we were able to check into the hotel that Schwabe had booked for us. The next day, we were picked up at the hotel, driven to Schwabe's headquarters, which was located on, of all places, *Willmar-Schwabe Strasse*. We were given a deluxe tour. Their facilities were immaculate and we were most impressed with their patented process of procuring, refining, and extracting a highly purified and concentrated form of Ginkgo biloba extract. We summoned the courage to ask for money to conduct a clinical trial in the U.S. They politely said no, but that they would be able to donate some Ginkgo tablets that we could use in our study. We thanked them immensely, and returned back to the U.S. ready to conquer the world. In order to attract funding, we would need to conduct a small pilot study to show that we knew how to do clinical research and to see if the product worked. With IRB approval from Liberty University, two students who needed internship credit, 40 senior citizen volunteers from my church, free Ginkgo from Schwabe, and a wing and a prayer, we conducted our first six-week clinical trial. The results were impressive and we were proud that we knew what we were doing. The next step now would be to publish our findings so that maybe, just maybe, Schwabe, or some other company, would agree to provide funding for a larger clinical trial. The results of our pilot study would indeed justify the need for a much larger trial; our results were published in *The Journal of Alternative and Complementary Medicine*.[2]

It worked! Shortly after publishing our results we submitted a proposal to Schwabe for a much larger clinical trial that would involve 262 healthy seniors over the age of 60. They agreed and would provide $150,000.00 for the new study. We asked for an additional $50,000, which they also agreed to provide through their U.S. subsidiary: "Nature's Way" of Springville, Utah. The $200,000.00 was, and still is, the largest grant ever awarded to Liberty University for clinical research. Schwabe had one condition: we would have to enroll at least 262 participants in the study. We agreed. We had one condition as well: we would have to be free to report our findings, whatever they may be, for better or for worse, good or bad. If Ginkgo worked, we would report it; if not, we needed to be free to report that as well. They agreed.

We screened over 500 participants and enrolled 262 (not 261 or 263, but 262) healthy senior citizens over the age of 60 in our study that would last six weeks. Each person received 60 mg Ginkgo or placebo to be taken three times a day for the six weeks. Each person received a battery of 13 separate neuropsychological assessment tests at the beginning and at the conclusion of the trial. By treatment end, the group that received the Ginkgo showed improvement in 11 of the 13 tests compared to those that received the placebo; and three were statistically significant. The improvement was modest, approximately 7-8%, but it was there, nevertheless, and it was primarily in the area known as speed of processing which meant that when asked to complete a paper and pencil task, those taking the Ginkgo were able to complete it significantly faster after the six weeks compared to the placebo group. It worked! We published our results in the journal: *Human Psychopharmacology: Clinical and Experimental,* and we had, indeed, conquered the world! We had confirmed what other researchers before us and since have found: Ginkgo biloba (at least the particular extract EGb-761® made by Schwabe Pharmaceutical Company of Karlsruhe, Germany) indeed works! The student who started everything with his question,

"Does *Ginkgo* work?" had since graduated, married, and had a child, but I was now finally able to give him an answer: "Yes, Ginkgo works!"

Figure10: Letter of Invitation from Schwabe Pharmaceutical Company of Karlsruhe, Germany, Inviting Me to Tour Their Facilities.

Dr. Willmar Schwabe
Arzneimittel

FAX TRANSMISSION

Dr Joseph Mix
Department of Health Sciences
Liberty University
Lynchburg, Virginia 24506-800
USA

Fax No 001/804 582 2554

Ihre Zeichen/Nachricht vom	Unsere Zeichen Dr Hoe/rs	Tel.-Durchwahl (07 21) 40 05- 492	Datum November 7, 1997

Postadresse:
Postfach 41 09 25
76209 Karlsruhe

Haus-/Lieferadresse
Willmar-Schwabe-Str. 4
76227 Karlsruhe

Telefon (07 21) 40 05 - 0
Telefax (07 21) 40 05 - 333

Clinical Research Department

Dear Doctor Mix,

Thank you for your letter of October 15 to Dr. Eaves. We appreciate your interest in our Ginkgo biloba special extract EGb 761 and your intention to conduct a study with this preparation.

I am sure it will not be a problem for us to provide you with the placebo tablets and suitable bottles. Moreover, we would be glad to meet you and discuss with you the research project outlined in your letter. We are very interested to learn more about your research and maybe we can help you with detailed information on our product and the extensive research that has already been done. So we will be happy to invite you to Karlsruhe. We would be delighted to show you our facilities and give you the opportunity to talk with all the people involved in Ginkgo biloba research for years.

I will try and call you the week after next, when I am back from a one-week vacation.

Looking forward to talking with you soon,

Sincerely yours

DR WILLMAR SCHWABE GMBH & CO
KARLSRUHE

Dr med Robert Hoerr
Senior Project Advisor

10 Additional Herbs that Heal

Garlic

Garlic, known for its strong odor, has long been prized for its culinary value, but is capable of demonstrating tremendous therapeutic potential as well. The chemical compound, *allicin*, found in garlic is thought to be largely responsible for its ability to reduce the risk of heart disease, lower cholesterol, lower blood pressure, and reduce the risks of certain types of cancer, particularly stomach and colorectal. Garlic has been referred to as "nature's antibiotic" for its anti-bacterial, antiviral, and antifungal properties.[3]

Garlic's ability to lower the risk of heart disease is thought to be the combination of several factors including its ability to prevent the agglutination of blood platelets, its ability to lower LDL cholesterol and possibly raise the HDL cholesterol, and its antihypertensive effect.[4] Probably, garlic's greatest contribution to lowering the risk of heart disease, however, is derived from its ability to prevent the *oxidation* of LDL cholesterol.[5]

Garlic was also effective in preventing the common cold, reducing recovery time, and reducing the duration of symptoms in a three-month study of 146 volunteers. The number of episodes of the common cold during the three-month study was significantly less in the treatment group compared to the placebo group (24 for those taking garlic vs. 65 for those taking placebo), as was the *duration* of symptoms (1.52 days for those taking garlic versus 5.01 days for those taking placebo). The average recovery period for those taking garlic was 4.63 days compared to 5.63 days for the placebo group.[6]

As the active ingredient in garlic, allicin, is inactivated upon cooking, fresh garlic is thought to be superior. One to two fresh cloves per day, or the equivalent, are recommended to obtain all the therapeutic benefits of this magnificent herb.

Milk Thistle

A little knowledge is a dangerous thing! In the previous chapter I cautioned you against the use of vitamin B_3 (niacin) in large doses due to its toxic effect on the liver. What I didn't mention was how I learned this: I failed to heed my own advice and almost destroyed my liver in the process. I didn't know. What I *did* know was that niacin could lower my cholesterol and that my cholesterol was high, so I figured if a little niacin is good, then more must be better, right? Wrong. I took upwards of 3 grams of niacin per day for several months after which a routine blood test revealed that my liver enzymes (ALT and AST) were elevated indicating that some damage had been done. I stopped the niacin and started taking an herb known as milk thistle. Today, my liver enzymes are normal!

Milk thistle actually promotes the regeneration of *hepatocytes* (liver cells). This actually allows the liver to heal itself. It is indicated for use in the treatment of liver ailments, including detoxification and cirrhosis associated with chronic alcohol abuse and viral hepatitis. The active ingredient is known as *silymarin* which is a very powerful antioxidant that may also protect the gallbladder and kidneys and is useful in cases of mushroom poisoning as well.[7] A typical therapeutic dose for liver problems is 140 mg of silymarin taken twice daily.

Black Elder

Rita was our neighbor when we lived in Italy. She was born and raised in Italy and had married an American man who had been stationed in her hometown. When his tour of duty was up, he left for the states and promised to come back for her once he was "settled." He never returned. She would go to the airport once a week, certain that he would be on the weekly flight from the U.S., but he never showed up. She was a delightful lady and never gave up hope that he would return for her though it had been many years without so much as a word from him. Rita spoke fluent English and Italian and would, on occasion, invite us to her house for a meal. I remember one such occasion when she invited my wife and me to her house for "a little lasagna." She greeted us at the door and welcomed us to be seated in her formal dining room (which she assured us was only used for special occasions). We started with hors d'oeuvres, then some antipasto, then some pasta, and then the lasagna. But we were not through. Then came the meat and the veal and the chicken and on and on until we thought we would explode (one didn't dare say "no" to Rita). Finally, after feeding as much as I could to Stella (her cocker spaniel) under the table, she brought out the "sambuca," a strong liqueur made from the berry of the European Black Elder (*Sambucus nigra*). She said it was good for our digestion and, since we couldn't say no to Rita, we gave it a try. Nagasaki and Hiroshima came to mind; we staggered home so glad that we only lived next door!

Sambucus nigra, in addition to making a strong after dinner liqueur, is an exciting herb used for relief from symptoms related to the common cold and the flu. The safety and effectiveness of oral Elderberry extract syrup (15 ml) for treating the flu were tested in a double blind, placebo-controlled trial involving 60 patients, aged 18-54 who reported influenza-like symptoms for up to 48 hours. The participants took the Elderberry syrup or placebo syrup four times daily for five days, and recorded the level and intensity of their flu symptoms. Analysis revealed that symptoms subsided, on average, four days sooner in those taking the Elderberry syrup.[8]

Only fully ripe (purple) berries should be used as the unripe (red) berries can be toxic. Elder interferes with the intestinal absorption of iron and should, therefore, should not be taken together. Sambucus should not be used by diabetics.

Myrrh

Yes, this is the same myrrh as in "gold, frankincense and myrrh" that was presented as a gift to the Christ child. Myrrh is an herbal product, but it is technically not an herb. It is the resin that exudes from incisions in the bark of *Commiphora myrrha*, a small tree native to Ethiopia, Somalia, and the Arabian peninsula.[9] Myrrh is prepared as a tincture and is used to treat sores of the mouth and throat, including canker sores, aphthous ulcers, and sore throat. I use it extensively in my dental practice to treat all of the above as well as generalized stomatitis, gingivitis, sores from ill-fitting dentures, trauma to the mouth caused by aspirin, hot liquids or hot foods, post-operative trauma, trauma from orthodontic braces, cheek biting, etc. It is my "ace in the hole" for soft tissue lesions. For hard tissue (teeth and bone) pain caused by decay or osteitis (dry socket), I employ another herbal product: *eugenol* (oil of cloves), which works equally as well.

Although capsules of the powdered resin have been prepared for internal use in the treatment of elevated cholesterol and triglyceride levels, there is insufficient evidence at this time to justify such use. It should only be used *topically* in the treatment of irritations to the mucous membranes of the mouth and throat. The undiluted tincture is applied directly to the sore with a cotton-tipped applicator (Q-tip®) two to three times daily. For sore throat, a gargle may be made by adding 5-10 drops of the tincture to one glass of water.[10] The patient is instructed to gargle and expectorate so as not to swallow. Women who are pregnant and women who are breastfeeding are cautioned against taking this product internally, as are diabetics since it has been shown to interfere with antidiabetic medication.[11]

Relatively speaking, the U.S. has been late to appreciate the value of herbal medicines, which have always been held in high esteem in oriental countries and Europe. But that is beginning to change as many U.S. consumers and scientists alike have come to recognize the tremendous therapeutic benefits that many herbs have to offer.

Table 12A: Several Medicinal Herbs; Uses, Dosages, and Cautions.

HERBS	MEDICAL PARTS	USES
Ginkgo biloba	leaves	enhances cognitive function, especially speed of processing
Garlic	garlic bulb	lowers cholesterol, lowers blood pressure, decreases risk of heart disease, antibiotic; may reduce risk of certain cancers and the common cold
Milk Thistle	ripe seeds	liver problems
Black Elder	fully ripe (purple) berries	cough, bronchitis, fever, colds, flu
Myrrh	myrrh is the resin that oozes from incisions in the bark of Commiphora myrrha	stomatitis, canker sores, aphthous ulcers, gingivitis, sore throat; for topical use only

DEFICIENCY	TOXICITY
high blood pressure; kidney stones; osteoporosis	extraction process needed to concentrate sufficient quantities of flavone glycosides and terpene lactones and to eliminate the highly allergenic ginkgolic acid; not to be taken by persons with high blood pressure or those taking blood thinning medication.
irregular heart beat (arrhythmias); atherosclerosis	the blood-thinning properties of garlic can cause bleeding. Headache and allergies have been reported. Offensive odor (due to sulfur-containing compounds) is a problem.
anemia	safe; no toxic side effects reported. Do not take with metronidazole.
anemia, aneurisms?, elevated cholesterol	use only fully ripe berries. unripe (red) berries may be toxic; should not be taken by diabetics; blocks the absorption of iron
delayed growth	hypoglycemic activity; should not be taken internally, especially if diabetic, or during pregnancy or lactation.

Flaxseed

"Wherever flaxseeds become a regular food item among the people, there will be better health."

Mahatma Gandhi[12]

Oil made from the flaxseed is one of the richest sources of omega-3 fatty acids. As such, it possesses heart-healthy properties, which include lowering LDL cholesterol (similar to the cholesterol-lowering effects of fish oil), inhibiting platelet aggregation, anti-inflammatory effects (remember, heart disease is largely an inflammatory process). Flaxseed oil does not appear to lower blood pressure.

Flaxseed reduced LDL cholesterol levels significantly compared with sunflower seeds in a double-blind, cross-over trial; HDL cholesterol levels were not affected.[13] Flaxseed has also been shown to improve glucose tolerance (decrease insulin resistance) in patients diagnosed with *metabolic syndrome*.[14] Metabolic syndrome, also known as *Syndrome X* or *Insulin Resistance Syndrome* is characterized by one or more of the following:

- obesity, primarily central obesity (apple, not pear-shaped)
- low HDL cholesterol
- high triglyceride levels
- hypertension
- glucose intolerance

Animal research has supported the anticancer effects of flaxseed and human trials suggest, though were not conclusive, that dietary flaxseed has the potential to reduce tumor size in breast cancer patients.[15] Finally, because flaxseed absorbs up to eight times its own weight in water, it promotes peristalsis, has a laxative effect and may also reduce bloat.[16] Its role, if any, in the prevention of colorectal cancer has not been determined. Flaxseeds aggravate diverticular disease (trust me on this!), therefore, for those prone to diverticulitis the oil should be used rather than the seed; one to two tablespoons full per day are recommended.[17] Oxygen, heat and light tend to be very destructive to this oil (not the seed), therefore, it cannot be used in cooking and should be kept refrigerated in opaque closed containers.

Green Tea

The Chinese have recognized the therapeutic value of tea for several thousand years; entire volumes could be devoted to the health benefits of *Camellia sinesis* from which both green tea and black tea are made. Green tea is produced by steaming the fresh-cut leaf; black tea is made by allowing the leaves to dry resulting in oxidation. Powerful antioxidant compounds known as polyphenols are the primary active ingredients in green tea and are largely responsible for its medicinal properties. Oxidation, which occurs in black tea inactivates many of these polyphenols. Because the steaming process used in the preparation of green tea preserves the polyphenol compounds, the anti-oxidant activity of green tea is six times greater than that of black tea.[18]

The primary health benefits derived from green tea are in the prevention of cancer and heart disease. The types of cancer that green tea has been shown to prevent include cancer of the stomach, bladder, colon, esophagus, lung, and pancreas. The apparent mechanism by which green tea prevents heart disease is through its ability to prevent the oxidation of LDL cholesterol and *foam cell* formation.[19] Green tea has also been shown to:

- Prevent tooth decay; mouthwashes made with green tea have been shown to decrease dental plaque formation and inhibit the growth of the cavity causing bacteria *Streptococcus mutans*.[20]
- Possess anti-inflammatory properties.

- Promote the growth of "good bacteria" in the intestine such as *Lactobacillus* and *Bifidobacter*.

- Inhibit the growth of "bad bacteria" in the intestine such as *Clostridium perfringens* and *Clostridium difficile*.

- Help protect the liver.

- Inhibit the enzyme xanthine oxidase (involved in the conversion of purines to uric acid), which contributes to the painful arthritic condition *gout*. The action of green tea in the prevention of gout was found to be similar to the anti-gout medication, allopurinol.[21]

- Reduce the incidence of Type 2 diabetes.[22]

- Reduce the risk of stroke.

- Assist with the oxidation of fat, therefore, it may be useful for the treatment of obesity.

The polyphenols in green tea are available in 100 mg, 150 mg, 175 mg, 333 mg and 500 mg capsules. A standard dose of 300-400 mg of polyphenols is recommended. Three cups of green tea normally contains between 240 and 320 mg polyphenols. Because green tea also contains anywhere from 10-50 mg caffeine per cup, restlessness and agitation may occur, so the capsules, since they do not contain caffeine may be preferred, especially for those who are pregnant or breastfeeding. Concurrent use with anticoagulants is not recommended.

Ginger

Ginger has traditionally been used primarily for nausea, vomiting, and motion sickness. Oral ginger 1 gram daily for four days was significantly more effective than placebo in the treatment of pregnancy-induced nausea and vomiting in women of less than 17 weeks gestation in a randomized, double-blind, placebo-controlled trial of 70 women.[23] Other studies investigating ginger's role to ameliorate chemotherapy-induced nausea have proved inconclusive.

The root (technically, ginger is not a root; it is a *rhizome*, or underground stem) also appears to demonstrate anti-inflammatory properties and has been used in the treatment of osteoarthritis (OA) and rheumatoid arthritis (RA). In a preliminary study involving 28 patients with rheumatoid arthritis and 18 patients with osteoarthritis, 74 % of the patients with RA and 55% of the patients with OA reported "marked" improvement in pain after taking 1-2 grams of powdered ginger per day for up to 2.5 years. With regard to swelling, 59% of RA patients, and 50% of OA patients reported "marked" improvement. No adverse events were reported. Since the study was based solely on self-report data, controlled and blinded studies are needed.[24]

Additional health benefits attributed to ginger root include:

- The reduction in the risk of heart disease (due to ginger's ability to decrease platelet aggregation).

- The reduction in the incidence and severity of migraine headaches (also due to ginger's "blood-thinning" effect).

- Antioxidant and immune system stimulating effects.

- Antimicrobial effects.[25]

No health hazards or side effects with the proper use of ginger are known. Recommended dosages are 1 gram of the powdered root per day. Cardiac arrhythmia and CNS depression may result from over dosage; gastric irritation and allergic reaction have been reported.

Saw Palmetto

Saw palmetto consists of the partially dried, ripe fruit of a low, bushy palm that grows from South Carolina to Florida. First recognized in Europe, it has been shown to relieve the symptoms of BPH (benign prostatic hyperplasia) by:

- Increasing urinary flow.

- Increasing ease of urination.

- Facilitating a more complete emptying of the bladder.

- Decreasing frequency of urination.[26]

Though some recent studies report conflicting results, a review of 18 randomized trials conducted between 1983 and 1997 and involving approximately 3000 participants concluded that saw palmetto herbal products provided some benefit in controlling lower urinary tract symptoms and flow measures in men with BPH.[27] The mechanism of action of saw palmetto is thought to be through its ability to block hormone (testosterone and estrogen) receptor sites and its anti-inflammatory effects. The recommended dose is 1-2 grams of the herb per day or 320 mg of an alcohol extract per day. It should be noted that saw palmetto is good for *symptomatic* relief of BPH only as it does not shrink the size of the enlarged prostate, nor does it play any role in the treatment of prostate cancer. Routine prostate screenings including digital palpation and blood tests for PSA should be conducted on a regular basis as advised by a qualified physician. Due to its ability to block hormone receptor sites, it should *not* be taken by patients receiving hormone therapy, nor should it be taken by those receiving anticoagulant medication.

Chaste Tree

Vitex agnus-castus is a bush or small tree that is native to the Mediterranean region and is seen as far as western Asia. A concentrated alcohol extract made from the dried and ripe fruit (berries) has been used extensively in Europe, particularly in Germany, for the treatment of gynecological disorders such as PMS, dysmenorrhea, and menopause. In menopause, estrogen production drops to about 10% of it premenopausal levels (it does not drop to zero during menopause since the adrenal gland continues to produce the hormone DHEA which is converted to estrogen). Progesterone production, however, drops to zero resulting in the characteristics of menopause: hot flashes, night sweats, mood swings, depression and osteoporosis. The mechanism by which the chaste tree berry extract helps to relieve these menopausal symptoms is not known.[28]

Chaste tree extract was effective in women with PMS (diagnosed according to the DSM III criteria) in a randomized, placebo-controlled trial. 170 women (average age 36 years) with PMS symptoms were given supplements of either 20 mg *Vitex agnus-castus* extract or placebo by mouth daily for three menstrual cycles. Improvements in irritability, and mood alteration were reported by 52% of those taking the extract, compared to 24% for the placebo group.[29]

Similarly, an extract of chaste berry was found to be effective in treating moderate to severe PMS in a prospective cohort study of 118 women with a mean age of 29.7 years. 67.8% of the women reported the severity of their symptoms consistently lessened by treatment end (three menstrual cycles). Seven participants discontinued chaste berry due to side effects; no serious adverse events were reported. Itching and rash were the most frequent complaints.[30]

Several mechanisms have been proposed to account for the ability of chaste berry to relieve the symptoms of PMS. Most agree that it inhibits the release of prolactin by the pituitary; some suggest that it increases levels of progesterone. Recommended dose is 30-40 mg of the concentrated alcohol extract per day.

Echinacea

Native Americans have known about and used this immune-boosting herb for a long time and it was common practice to treat respiratory infections by holding a piece of the dried root of *Echinacea angustafolia* in the mouth. There are several *Echinacea* species that are used today with the most common being *Echinacea purpurea*. Known as the purple coneflower the aerial parts (stem, leaves, and flower) are more frequently utilized and have been more thoroughly researched than the root portions of this or other species.

Echinacea acts as an immune stimulant thought to occur as a result of its ability to increase phagocytic activity and cell-mediated immunity by stimulating the production of lymphocytes, macrophages, mononuclear cells and killer cells.[31] Echinacea also demonstrated direct bactericidal activity which was found to approximate that of vancomycin.[32]

Though some studies have failed to show its effectiveness, the majority of studies indicate that *Echinacea* is effective for the treatment of upper respiratory infections, flu-like infections, and for reducing the severity and length of symptoms accompanying the common cold. Several studies offer cases in point:

- In a 2005 study, Echinilin®, a formulation prepared from freshly harvested *Echinacea pupurea* plants was found to be effective for the treatment of the common cold. For a seven day period, volunteers took either Echinilin® or placebo at the onset of their cold, with eight doses (5 ml/dose) on day one, and three doses on subsequent days. Those in the treatment group experienced a more significant decrease in the total number of symptoms, suggesting that Echinilin® may have led to faster resolution of the cold symptoms.[33]

- An earlier study of 282 subjects showed that the same preparation, Echinilin® produced lower daily symptom scores than placebo. The subjects, aged 18-65 years with a history of two or more colds in the previous year, were randomly assigned to take Echinilin® or placebo at the onset of the first cold symptom, consuming 10 doses the first day and 4 doses daily on subsequent days for seven days. Total daily symptom scores were lower by 23.1% in the Echinacea group than in placebo.[34]

- The ability of *Echinacea* purpurea to prevent infection with rhinovirus type 39 (RV-39) was tested in a randomized, double blind, placebo-controlled clinical trial. 48 previously healthy adults were administered Echinacea or placebo. 2.5 ml three times per day for seven days before and seven days after intranasal inoculation with RV-39. Colds developed in 58% of patients in the Echinacea group and 82% in the placebo group, which was not found to be statistically significant.35

PLAY YOUR HAND WELL

- A 2000 study that used Echinacea Plus®, an herbal tea preparation containing *Echinacea purpurea* and *Echinacea angustafolia*, decreased the duration of symptoms of cold or flu when taken at early onset of symptoms. The trial was double blind, placebo-controlled, and involved 95 subjects aged 24-62 years. Symptom relief, number of days of symptoms, and number of days before noticeable symptom change were significantly improved in the Echinacea Plus group compared to the placebo group.[36]

- *Echinacea* demonstrated effective symptom relief for viral respiratory tract infections in a double blind, placebo-controlled, multicenter study. Symptom relief response time was reduced in the Echinacea group compared to placebo.[37]

- Echinagard® shortened the course of upper respiratory infections in a double blind, placebo-controlled study involving 120 patients randomized to either Echinagard® or placebo. Median improvement was reported in four days for the Echinagard® group compared to eight days for the placebo group.[38]

- A double blind, placebo-controlled study showed that *Echinacea* taken at the onset of upper respiratory symptoms was able to reduce the duration of the illness by 25% to 33%.[39]

Several of these studies underscore the importance of taking the *Echinacea* as early as possible at the very first sign of developing cold symptoms. A typical dose would be 15-30 drops of the alcohol extract, two to five times per day. The alcohol extract (tincture) is preferred to the capsules since it may stimulate oral lymphatic tissue as a result of direct contact with the mouth (Indians knew this a long time ago which is why they would hold the root in their mouths for a time!). Echinacea should not be used for more than eight consecutive weeks at a time.

Table 12B: Several Medicinal Herbs; Uses, Dosages, and Cautions.

HERBS	MEDICAL PARTS	USES
Flax	oil from seeds	anti-inflammatory, lowers LDL, reduces risk of heart disease, inhibits platelet aggregation
Green Tea	steamed, fresh cut leaves	prevention of cancer heart disease, tooth decay, gout, type 2 diabetes, and stroke, largely due to its powerful anti-oxidant properties
Ginger	root	used to treat nausea, vomiting and motion sickness; anti-inflammatory, anti-migraine; stimulates immune system; inhibits platelet aggregation
Saw Palmetto	dried, ripe fruit	symptoms associated with BPH (benign enlarged prostate) and chronic bladder infections
Chaste Tree	dried, ripe berries	PMS, dysmenorrheal, menopause
Echinacea	aerial, overground parts (stem, leaves, flower) and the root	immune booster used to treat upper respiratory infections, common cold, and flu

DEFICIENCY	TOXICITY
1-2 tablespoonfuls per day	laxative effect
300-400 mg polyphenols per day from capsules or tea (3 cups)	pregnancy and breastfeeding due to caffeine content; interferes with anticoagulants
1 gram/day of the powdered root in capsule form	cardiac arrhythmia, CNS depression; increased risk of bleeding. Some advocate that it should not be used in pregnancy or lactation. May cause stomach irritation; do not take on an empty stomach; allergic reaction possible.
anemia, aneurisms?, elevated cholesterol	use only fully ripe berries. unripe (red) berries may be toxic; should not be taken by diabetics; blocks the absorption of iron
delayed growth	hypoglycemic activity; should not be taken internally, especially if diabetic, or during pregnancy or lactation.
15-30 drops of the alcohol extract, 2-5 times per day	allergy; should not be used for more than 8 consecutive weeks

CHAPTER 9

THE MIX FOOD QUALITY INDEX™ AND THE TOP 10 FOODS

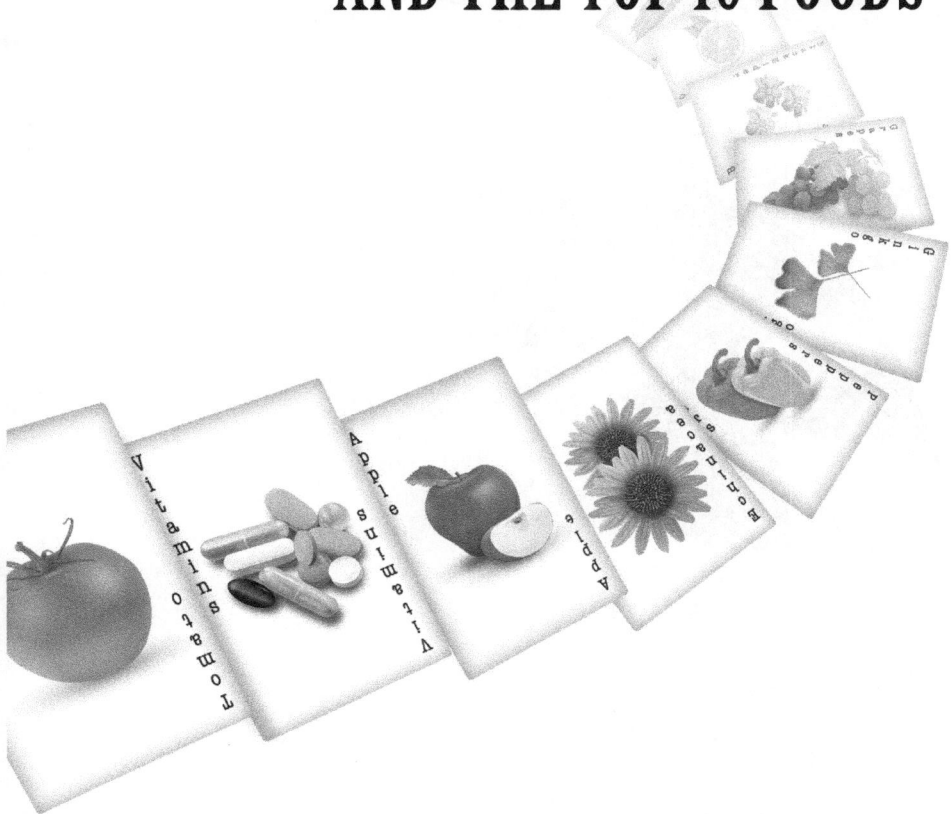

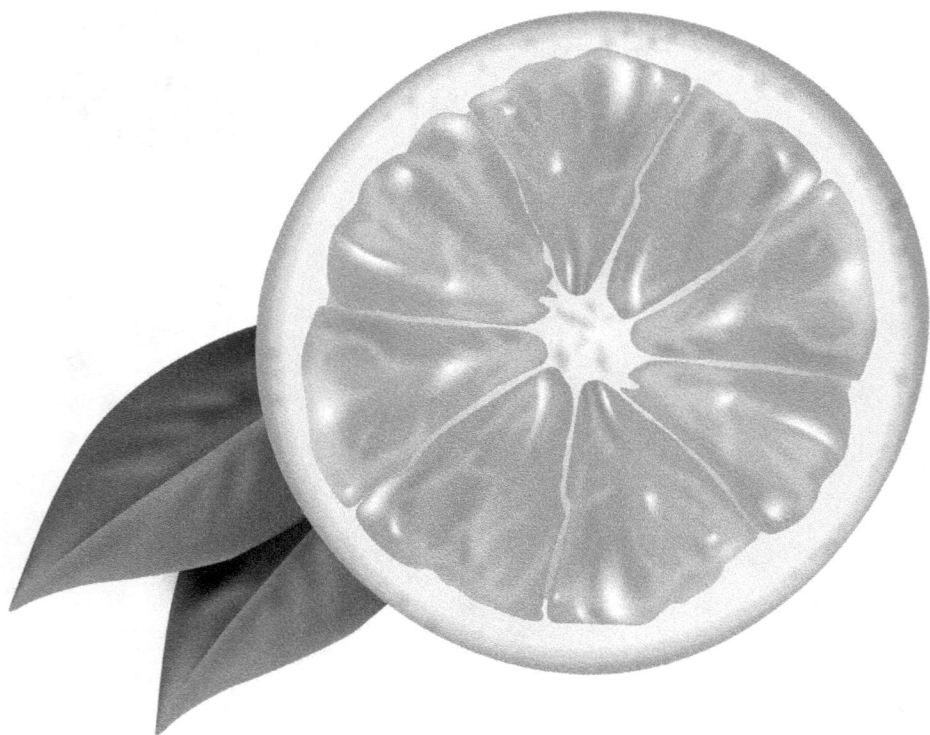

While attempting to come up with my top 10 list of the most nutritious foods of all time, it occurred to me that there should be an objective means to assess food quality; a standardized rubric by which various foods could be compared, rated and scored that would take into account their healthy and not-so-healthy qualities. Unable to locate such a measure, I proceeded to create what I have called the "Mix Food Quality Index™." The concept is simple: various nutrient indicators associated with healthy and non-healthy events are chosen and foods are rated and scored as to the extent to which they either have or do not have those particular indicators. The presence of "healthy" indicators *increases* the food's total score, while "unhealthy" indicators *decrease* that score.

The Mix Food Quality Index™ is an overall composite score which assesses the *positive* qualities of a particular food such as antioxidant potential, cardiovascular support, and protein delivery, as well as those *negative* qualities which may contribute to obesity, diabetes, high blood pressure, heart disease, and stroke. For the system to work and to permit valid comparison, energy (calories) must be controlled for, so that calculations are based on the quantity of the food capable of yielding 200 calories (kcal), which represents 10%, or 1/10th of a typical 2000-calorie daily intake. Standard nutritional analysis data is obtained from the USDA National Nutrient Database.[1] Amounts of the preselected nutrient indicators are recorded and percentages of the recommended adult intakes (as established by a recognized authority such as the Institute of Medicine or the World Health Organization) are calculated.

> *If a particular food provides 10% of your daily calo-*
> *ries, then it is reasonable to expect that it should also*
> *provide at least 10% of your beneficial nutrients. This*
> *is the basis for the Mix Food Quality Index ™.*

A score is then assigned according to the extent to which the food was able to deliver a minimum of 10% of a given nutrient. If a particular food provides 10% of your daily calories, then it is reasonable to expect that it should also provide at least 10% of your beneficial nutrients. This is the basis for the Mix Food Quality Index ™.

Scoring

If the food provides 10% or more of the recommended daily intake of a given nutrient, it receives the maximum score of 1 for that nutrient. Delivering greater than 10% of the nutrient does not rate a higher score; the scoring system is designed to identify foods capable of providing a broad range of nutrients and not reward a food simply because it provides 650% of vitamin C, for example. If the food provides less than 10% of the recommended daily intake, then it receives a score proportional to 1. For example, a food providing 4.5% of the daily-recommended intake of vitamin E would receive a score of 0.45. Once again, it is important to remember that calories are controlled for, and the quantity of the food used in the calculations will be that quantity necessary to yield 200 calories.

"Good" nutrients such as the antioxidant vitamins, beneficial minerals, "good" fatty acids, and fiber are added together and will increase the overall score; "bad" nutrients such as saturated fat, trans fat, sugars, and fiber will be subtracted from the score. The final index score will then be an objective assessment of overall food quality (see Appendix for complete scoring of selected foods). There are four components to the Mix Index: the Antioxidant Potential Index (A.P.I.), the Cardiovascular Support Index (C.S.I.), the Protein Delivery Index (P.D.I.), and the Not-in-the-Interest-of-Health Index (N.I.H.); the Final Mix Food Quality Score = the sum of the first three components minus the last.

$$\textit{The Mix Food Quality Index}^{TM} = (API + CSI + PDI) - NIH$$

The Antioxidant Potential Index (API)

The importance of antioxidants in protecting against damage from free radicals has already been mentioned. The first step in calculating the food quality index is to determine the antioxidant potential of a food as determined by the presence of four powerful antioxidant indicators: vitamin C, beta-carotene, vitamin E, and the mineral, selenium. Recommendations from the Institute of Medicine[2] and Dr. Ken Cooper[3] have set the recommended levels of these antioxidants at 90 mg, 15 mg (from *food* only, *not* supplements), 15 mg, and 55 mcg per day respectively. Food quantities equivalent to 200 calories were selected, percentages calculated, and each food was scored according to the format mentioned above. See the example of how to score the API for the onion and the sweet potato in Tables 14-18; the rest of the scoring may be seen in the Appendix. Not surprisingly, spinach and broccoli, each scored a perfect four out of four for their abilities to deliver all four antioxidant indicators in quantities greater than 10% of recommended levels. Carrot and tomato came in third and fourth due to their low levels of selenium. M&Ms and french fries brought up the bottom of the list with little or no antioxidant potential.

The Cardiovascular Support Index (CSI)

The indicators chosen to assess cardiovascular health were *calcium* and *potassium* (for their abilities to reduce blood pressure), *magnesium* (for its role in the proper functioning of the heart muscle), the "good" fats, *omega-3* and *monounsaturated* (for their LDL cholesterol lowering effects), and *fiber* (also, for its ability to lower cholesterol). As with antioxidant potential, amounts were recorded (after controlling for calories), and percentages compared with the recommended intakes established by the Institute of Medicine and the WHO.[4] See Tables 14-18 for scoring; other scores in the Appendix. Spinach, soybean, and flaxseed topped the list, with soybean scoring a perfect six out of six for its ability to provide all heart-healthy indicators in quantities greater than 10%. The hot dog finished last.

The Protein Delivery Index (PDI)

Protein is important for building and repairing muscle tissue (which includes muscles, tendons, ligaments, bones, teeth, and connective tissues), for the hemoglobin that red blood cells need to transport oxygen, for neurotransmitters, hormones, and for a healthy immune system. The World Health Organization estimates that 10-15% of daily caloric intake should come from protein. Protein differs in *quantity* as well as *quality*. As discussed in Chapter 3, animal protein from milk, eggs, fish, beef is of *high* quality because it contains all the essential amino acids. With the exception of soybeans, most plant protein does not contain all essential amino acids and is of a lower quality. Of the several methods used to evaluate protein quality: the PER (Protein Efficiency Ratio), the BV (Biological Value), the AAS (Amino Acid Score), and the PDCAAS (Protein Digestibility Corrected Amino Acid Score), the latter has been adopted by the U.S. Food and Drug Administration and the World Health Organization as the preferred method.[5] All methods involve comparing the amino acid profile of the protein in question to that of a standard such as pure egg white (which receives the highest score of 1.0).

For scoring purposes, I use a simplified *estimate* of the PDCAAS, which appears in Table 13.[6]   As expected, animal protein came out on top with chicken, egg, and salmon all receiving perfect scores of 2.0. Soybean, peanuts, corn, and wheat germ were the highest scorers for plant protein; broccoli, spinach, flaxseed and almonds received honorable mention in this category. The scores are presented in Tables 14-18 and in the Appendix.

Table 13. Estimated PDCAAS Scores for Various Foods.

FOOD	PDCAAS (Estimate)
Egg white	1
Ground beef	1
Chicken	1
Tuna	1
Soybeans	0.9
Legumes	0.6
Peanuts	0.5
Grains	0.4
Nuts and seeds	0.4
Broccoli	0.3
Spinach	0.3
Other vegetables	0.2
Fruit	0.1

The Not-in-the-Interest-of-Health Index (NIH)

This is the final component of the overall Mix Food Quality Index ™ and it is used to assess the presence of *unhealthy* indicators in certain foods that are associated with high blood pressure, heart disease, obesity, and diabetes. The unhealthy indicators used in this index are saturated fat, trans fat, sodium and sugars. The term *sugars* refers to all simple mono and disaccharide carbohydrates, both natural and added, found in a given food, and though some feel that "natural" sugars are not as "bad" as added sugar, sugar is still sugar no matter where it comes from and can contribute to some of the health problems listed above, hence it is included in this index. It should be noted that the recommended intakes of these indicators are the *maximum* levels recommended by the World Health Organization based on a 2000 calorie per day diet. These recommendations are tabulated in the Appendix. This contribution of each of the above unhealthy indicators is scored the same as the other indices; however, the sum is *subtracted* from the total to produce the final Food Quality Index score. Results are presented in Tables 14-18 and in the Appendix.

Now, It's Your Turn

I designed this index to assist you in making wise food choices. You can select any particular food that you wish and calculate its score to see how it compares to my top 10. You will notice blank spaces in the tables for you to write in your selected food. Now, follow these steps to score your favorite (or not-so-favorite) food:

Step 1:

Select a food item from the USDA Nutrient Database.

- The website is: http://www.nal.usda.gov/fnic/foodcomp/search/

Step 2:

Select the amount necessary to produce 200 calories.

- You will do this by "trial and error," increasing or decreasing the amount until you see the number "200" appear in the column of the analysis report labeled "Value per _____ grams."

● The row will be labeled "energy," and the units will be in kilocalories ("kcal").

Step 3:

Calculate the Antioxidant Potential Index (API).

● Scroll down the report and record the *values* for *vitamin C, beta-carotene, vitamin E* and *selenium* in the blanks provided in Table 14. Divide these numbers by their respective recommended intake levels (90 mg, 15 mg, 15 mg, and 55 mcg) to obtain *percentages* of the recommended levels.

● Note: beta-carotene values are usually given in micrograms (mcg) and the recommended intake is 15 milligrams (mg) so you will have to convert micrograms to milligrams by moving the decimal point three places to the left.

● 1 mg = 1000 mcg

● 1mcg = .001 mg

● Watch your units to make sure they match!

● Score each nutrient as follows:

  – If the percentage is 10% or greater, score a 1.0

  – If the percentage is less than 10%, score proportionately. For example: if a carrot yields 7% of vitamin C, then its score for that vitamin is 0.7. If another food yields 1% of vitamin E, then its score is 0.1

  – Sum the scores for the four nutrients.

● The result is the API.

● Use the scoring for the onion as an example and record in Table 14.

Step 4:

Calculate the Cardiovascular Support Index (CSI).

- Record the values for *calcium, potassium, magnesium, monounsaturated fatty acids, omega-3 fatty acids,* and *fiber.*

- Monounsaturated fatty acids will appear on the report as "Fatty acids, total, monounsaturated."

- Omega-3 fats will be labeled on the report as 18:3, 20:5 n-3, 22:5 n-3, and 22:6 n-3. Add these together to obtain the omega-3 fat total (some 18:3 fats are omega-6, but most are omega-3; also, the 20:5, 22:5, and 22:6 fats are the fish oils so unless you have chosen fish, these are likely to be zero).

- Fiber will be listed on the report as "Fiber, total dietary."

- As you did in Step 3, convert these amounts to percentages by dividing by the respective recommended intake levels of 1000 mg, 4700 mg, 370 mg, 15 grams, 4 grams, and 26 grams.

- Watch your units to make sure they match.

- Score as above, sum, and record the total in Table 15. This number is the CSI score (use the scoring for onion as a guide).

Step 5:

Calculate the Protein Delivery Index (PDI).

- Record protein *quantity* from report (located under "energy") and convert to a percentage by dividing by 75 grams (the recommended average daily adult intake based on 10-15% of a 2000 calorie per day diet).

- Record protein *quality* from Table 13.

- The sum is the PDI; record in Table 16.

Step 6:

Calculate the Not-in-the-Interest-of-Health Index (NIH).

- Record amounts for *total saturated fats, trans fats, total sugars,* and *sodium.*

- Trans fats will most likely be zero and may not be listed.

- Calculate percentages by dividing by 22 grams, 2 grams, 50 grams, and 1500 mg respectively.

- Score as above and record in Table 17.

Step 7:

Calculate the Mix Food Quality Index ™.

- Add the API, CSI, and PDI together.

- Subtract the NIH.

- The result is the Mix Food Quality Index ™ score.

- Compare to my top 10 picks and other foods and enjoy!

Table 14. The Antioxidant Potential Index (API)

NUTRIENT	RA[1]	UNITS	ONION (500 grams/200 kcal)[2]		
			Amt.	% RA	Score
Vitamin C	90	mg	37.0	41.1	1
Beta-Carotene	15	mg	0	0	0
Vitamin E	15	mg	0.1	0.7	0.07
Selenium	55	mcg	2.5	4.5	0.45
TOTAL					1.52

Table 15. The Cardiovascular Health Index (CSI)

NUTRIENT	RA[1]	UNITS	ONION (500 grams/200 kcal)[2]		
			Amt.	% RA	Score
Calcium	1000	mg	115.0	11.5	1
Potassium	4700	mg	730.0	15.5	1
Magnesium	370	mg	50.0	13.5	1
MUFA[3]	15	g	0.1	0.7	0.07
Omega-3[4]	4	g	0	0	0
Fiber[5]	26	g	8.5	32.7	1
TOTAL					4.07

SWEET POTATO (233 grams/200 kcal)[2]			YOUR FOOD HERE		
Amt.	% RA	Score	Amt.	% RA	Score
5.6	6.2	0.62			
19.8	132.0	1			
0.6	4.0	0.40			
1.4	2.5	0.25			
		2.27			

SWEET POTATO (233 grams/200 kcal)[2]			YOUR FOOD HERE		
Amt.	% RA	Score	Amt.	% RA	Score
70.0	7.0	0.70			
785.0	16.7	1			
58.0	15.7	1			
0	0	0			
0	0	0			
7.0	26.9	1			
		3.70			

Table 16. The Protein Index (PDI)

NUTRIENT	RA[1]	UNITS	ONION (500 grams/200 kcal)[2]		
			Amt.	% RA	Score
Protein (Quantity)[6]	75	g	5.5	7.3	0.73
Protein (Quality)[7]	-	-			0.20
TOTAL					0.93

Table 17. The NIH Index (Not-in-the-Interest-of-Health Index)

NUTRIENT	RA[1]	UNITS	ONION (500 grams/200 kcal)[2]		
			Amt.	% RA	Score
SAT FAT[8]	22	g	0.2	0.9	0.09
TRANS FAT[9]	2	g	0	0	0
Sugars[10]	50	g	21.2	42.4	1
Sodium	1500	mg	20.0	1.3	0.13
TOTAL					1.22

[1]   Recommended adult daily intake as established by a recognized authority such as the Institute of Medicine or the World Health Organization (WHO). In cases where there are different recommendations for males and females, the two have been averaged together for the purpose of facilitating scoring. There is no RDA for beta-carotene; the recommendation of 15 mg per day is based on Dr. Kenneth Cooper's recommendation of 15 mg beta-carotene per day from food only (see references).

[2]   The scoring system is based on the quantity of food required to yield 200 calories (1/10th of a daily calorie intake of 2000).

[3]   Monounsaturated fatty acids.

[4]   Omega-3 fatty acids.

SWEET POTATO (233 grams/200 kcal)[2]			YOUR FOOD HERE		
Amt.	% RA	Score	Amt.	% RA	Score
3.66	4.8	0.48			
		0.20			
		0.68			

SWEET POTATO (233 grams/200 kcal)[2]			YOUR FOOD HERE		
Amt.	% RA	Score	Amt.	% RA	Score
0	0	0			
0	0	0			
9.7	19.4	1			
128.0	8.5	0.85			
		1.85			

5   Based on a 2000 calorie (kcal) per day diet and the WHO recommendation of 10-13 grams per 1000 calories.

6   Based on the WHO recommendation of 10-15% of daily calories for a 2000 calorie per day diet.

7   As assessed by estimates of the PDCAAS (Protein Digestibility Corrected Amino Acid Score). See Table 13.

8   Saturated Fat.

9   Trans Fat.

10   Based on the WHO recommendation of no more than 10% of calories per day from sugar for a 2000 calorie per day diet. Includes all sugars, natural and added.

Mix Food Quality Index ™ (Onion) = (1.52 + 4.07 + 0.93) – 1.22

                                           (API)   (CSI)   (PDI)   (NIH)

= **5.30** ← Write Final Index Score Here

Mix Food Quality Index ™ (Sweet Potato) = (2.27 + 3.70 + 0.68) – 1.85

                                           (API)   (CSI)   (PDI)   (NIH)

= **4.80** ← Write Final Index Score Here

Mix Food Quality Index ™ **(Your food)** = (_____ + _____ + _____) – _____

                                                        (API)   (CSI)   (PDI)   (NIH)

= ⬜ ⟵ Write Final Index
Score Here

Mix Food Quality Index ™ **(Your food)** = (_____ + _____ + _____) – _____

                                                        (API)   (CSI)   (PDI)   (NIH)

= ⬜ ⟵ Write Final Index
Score Here

My Top 10

The beauty of this system is that it evaluates foods for their potential to contribute to health as well as for their potential to detract from it, in an objective, standardized approach that permits comparison between various foods and facilitates wise food choices. I really enjoy scoring a new food to see how it compares with others and I have evaluated many, which you will find in the appendix to this book. Still, there are many that as yet have not been evaluated, so if you don't see your favorite "health" food among my top 10, then go ahead, crunch the numbers and see where it ranks. With this index, each food begins on a level playing field and is given an equal opportunity to "put up or shut up:" the food is delivering 10% of the calories, can it also deliver 10% of the nutrients? It bears repeating that delivering more than 10% does not earn it a higher score since we are more interested in the food's ability to provide a broad range of nutrients than we are in its ability to provide a great deal of one at the expense of the others. Finally, I would caution you into reading too much into any single component index (API, CSI, PI, or NIH); it is the final composite index score that takes into consideration all of the nutritive factors that really counts (see Table 18). Now, my top 10:

#10: Carrot

The index revealed that carrots are a *great source* of all the antioxidant vitamins, calcium, potassium, magnesium and fiber. It was *not* a good source of monounsaturated fatty acids (MUFAs), had no omega-3s and was only fair in terms of quantity and quality of its protein. Although there's nothing wrong with landing in the top 10, what really kept the carrot from ranking higher was its high sodium and sugar content. The high sugar content is the reason it has a high glycemic index (Chapter 2). Still #10 is not bad, so chomp away! By the way, the orange was close behind at #11.

#9: Almond

Almonds made an unbelievable "comeback" considering they got off to a rather slow start with a poor showing in the API. They scored very well in the CSI, due to their high MUFA, magnesium, and fiber content. They are also fair sources of calcium and potassium and, since they have so few negatives, they scored very well on the NIH. Now, the question is: would a walnut have score higher? Try it and see.

#8: Red Pepper

With more vitamin C than an orange, what did you expect? This red beauty did very well on the API and pretty well on the CSI, considering the fact that it has no fats. Although not known for protein, it did have some, and very few negatives (except high in sugar).

#7: Salmon

Why take fish oil capsules when you can have the real thing? Well, at least *plants* didn't take all the top 10 spots. Although salmon didn't do very well in the antioxidant category, it had enough going for it in other areas to secure a top spot. This fish, as you would expect, scored very well on the CSI and was the only food in the top 10 to receive a perfect score on the PDI.

#6: Tomato

A great source of all the antioxidants, except selenium. Tomatoes also scored very well in terms of cardiovascular support, have some protein and few negatives. Although not one of the indicators used in this system, tomatoes are an excellent source of the antioxidant *lycopene* which has greatly improved prostate health in men.

#5: Flaxseed

Who knew? Not much of an antioxidant, but its got everything else. It has no negatives. (on second thought if you suffer from diverticulosis, it does have a big negative; the seeds get stuck in those nasty little pouches and cause much aggravation, distress and discomfort). In that case you would need to take the flaxseed *oil* (easily spoils when exposed to light, heat, and oxygen so keep refrigerated in an opaque and airtight container; cannot be used for cooking). Flaxseed is one of the best sources of the heart healthy omega-3 fatty acids.

#4: Broccoli

I always think of my daughter, Becky, when I think of broccoli. For her third grade Sunday school's party to celebrate St. Patrick's Day, all the kids were asked to bring something *green*. Some brought green cupcakes, some brought cookies with green icing. Becky brought broccoli! Broccoli received a perfect score on the API, and is able to deliver more vitamin C than an orange! It is a great source of all the heart healthy indicators on the CSI except the good fats, has few negatives and its high protein content was a surprise.

#3: Wheat Germ

Wheat germ is an excellent source of vitamin E and is able to deliver protein in quantity as well as quality. It is also an excellent source of the antioxidant mineral, selenium (provided that the wheat was not grown in selenium poor soil). Wheat germ received the lowest score on the NIH (that's a good thing!) of any of the foods listed in the top 10.

#2: Soybean

When I began the scoring process, I was sure that soybean would come out on top, but second isn't all that bad! After a really slow start in the antioxidant category, the soybean came on really strong in delivering protein and was the only food to receive a perfect score on the CSI. It has the highest quality protein of any plant, rivaling the high-quality protein of eggs, fish, beef, and milk. In addition, soybean is an excellent source of *phytoestrogens*, which may help protect against breast cancer. Don't like tofu? I don't either, but it is good for you!

#1: Spinach

Popeye knew! Spinach blew the others out of the water and is pure dynamite when it comes to the ability to deliver nutrients. It's got it all. Spinach receives a perfect score when it comes to antioxidant potential and is great for the heart since 868 grams of spinach (which yields 200 calories) delivers 85.9%, 103%, and 185% of the adult daily requirements for calcium, potassium and magnesium respectively!! It also possesses a fair amount of protein and is a great source of *lutein* and *zeaxanthin*. Because of the presence of these two powerful antioxidants, spinach has been directly linked to an approximate 50% drop in age-related blindness.7 And Popeye didn't even know this; he was just eating it for the iron!

Well, there you have it: a system, which permits comparison of foods, based on their healthy and unhealthy characteristics. While the system does not take into account all factors (no system ever could), such as the presence of other antioxidant compounds like the *proanthocyanidins* found in grapes, it is an excellent screening tool to permit valid comparison, to facilitate healthy food choices, and is one more tool for your bag of tricks so you can play your hand better. Life is good!

Table 18: The Mix Food Quality Index™

FOOD ITEMS	API	CSI
Spinach	4.00	5.07
Soybean	1.57	6.00
Wheat Germ	2.00	4.73
Broccoli	4.00	4.31
Flaxseed	1.10	5.59
Tomato	3.00	4.20
Salmon	1.73	4.22
Red Pepper	3.11	3.45
Almond	1.16	4.44
Carrot	3.09	4.07
Orange	2.11	4.07
Cabbage	2.44	4.06
Peanut	1.45	3.85
Onion	1.52	4.07
Corn	1.45	3.58
Chicken (no skin)	1.13	2.77
Sweet Potato	2.27	3.70
Egg	1.93	2.84
White Potato (with skin)	1.16	3.26
Chicken (with skin)	1.27	2.70
Grape	1.49	2.83
Apple (with skin)	1.54	2.61
Hamburger	1.20	2.19
Hot Dog	0.98	1.75
French Fries	0.51	3.45
Candy (M&M's)	0.34	2.56

PLAY YOUR HAND WELL

PDI	NIH	Mix Food Quality Index™ Score
1.30	1.97	**8.40**
1.90	1.26	**8.21**
1.40	0.46	**7.67**
1.30	2.09	**7.52**
1.31	0.82	**7.18**
1.20	1.51	**6.89**
2.00	1.22	**6.73**
1.05	1.26	**6.35**
1.38	0.87	**6.11**
0.80	2.09	**5.87**
0.63	1.00	**5.81**
1.30	2.10	**5.70**
1.50	1.32	**5.48**
0.93	1.22	**5.30**
1.40	1.41	**5.02**
2.00	1.06	**4.84**
0.68	1.85	**4.80**
2.00	2.22	**4.55**
0.85	0.77	**4.50**
2.00	1.49	**4.48**
0.38	1.13	**3.57**
0.23	1.08	**3.30**
2.00	2.35	**3.04**
1.91	2.42	**2.22**
0.32	2.07	**2.21**
0.23	2.67	**0.46**

CHAPTER 10
: LIFE IS GOOD!

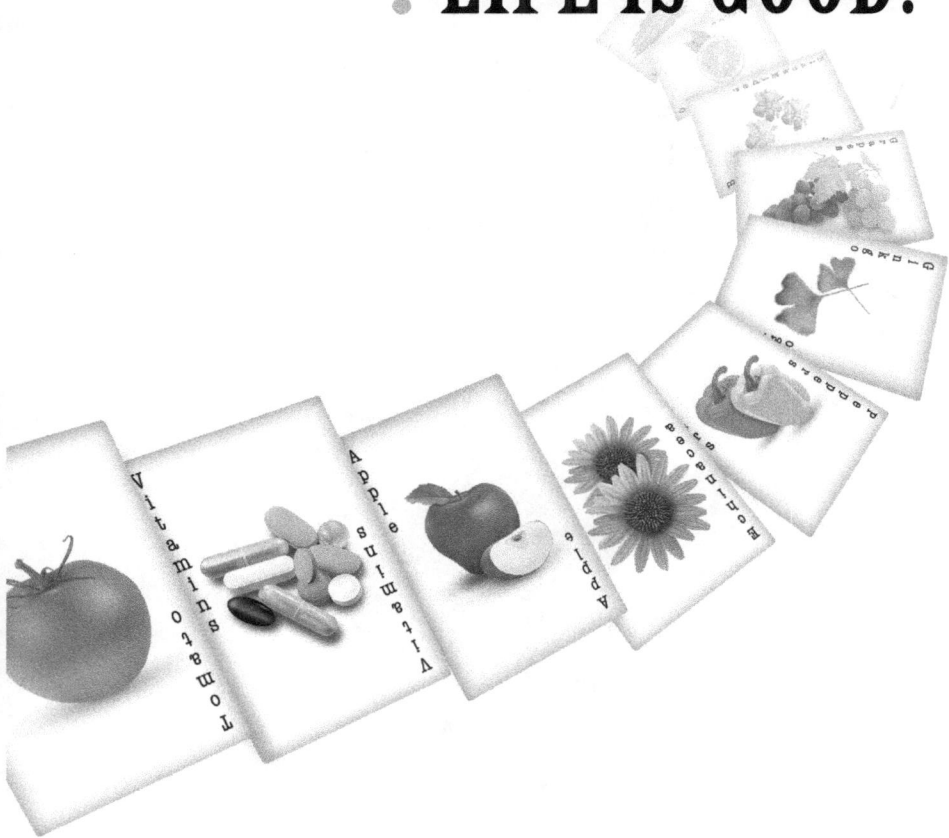

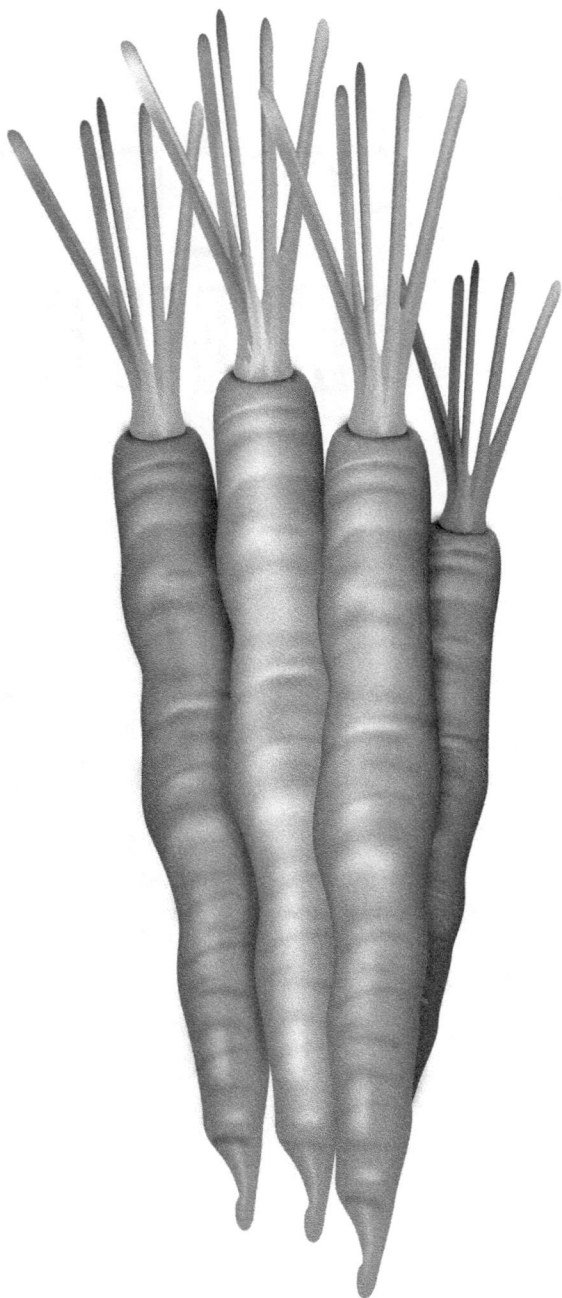

astly, but very importantly, know that life is good. Worry accomplishes nothing and switching from one new diet to another produces endless cycles of weight loss and weight gain that only makes matters worse. "Diets" rarely work. Instead, make wise food choices over the long run, through gradual changes in your eating habits. If you "mess" up, do not worry. Life is too short to punish yourself. A few final points to consider:

Exercise is Good.

My first car was a 1965 Volkswagen beetle. It had more rust than chrome and if you lifted up the floor mat on the passenger side, you could see the road underneath. It mostly sat idle, because I was afraid to drive it for fear it would break and fall apart. Thankfully, our bodies are not like that. They must be driven; they must be used. Exercise makes us *stronger*.

There are two types of exercise: *aerobic* and *anaerobic*. Aerobic means *with oxygen* and it is a type of low to moderate intensity exercise that is most beneficial for cardiovascular fitness. The key to aerobic exercise is to get your heart rate up to 60-80% of your maximum heart rate and keep it there for 30 minutes, five times a week (see the recommendations on exercise issued jointly by the American College of Sports Medicine and the American Heart Society in the Appendix). You can estimate your maximum heart rate by subtracting your age from the number 220. Examples of aerobic exercise are running, jogging, tennis, walking, etc. The key is to choose an activity that you enjoy and that will get your heart rate up and stick to it. The other type of exercise is anaerobic which means *without oxygen*. A good example of anaerobic activity is *weight training* which is an important component of a good, overall exercise program. In fact, for weight control, weight training is indispensible. Weight training builds muscle, and muscle burns calories and that really is the key to weight loss and keeping it off. Remember my 1965 beetle? It had a 4-cylinder engine and burned *some* fuel, but not nearly as much fuel as my friend's 8-cylinder Chrysler. With weight training, you can turn your 4-cylinder "Volkswagen" muscles into 6 or 8-cylinder "Chrysler," or even 12 cylinder "Jaguar" muscles, which will burn more fuel and facilitate weight loss.

When we lived in Italy, we drove a Fiat ("Fix it again, Tony") and an Alfa Romeo. The Fiat never ran, but the Alfa Romeo used two different types of fuel: regular *gasoline* and *propane* gas which was located in a tank in the trunk. If we ran out of gas while driving on the road, we would open the trunk, flip a switch and the car would then run on the propane. Our bodies are like that: we also have two types of fuel (except that we do not have a switch to flip in our trunks). The main fuel is *glycogen*, which is stored in the muscles and consists of long chains of glucose molecules. The other is *fat*. Glucose can be used to fuel aerobic or anaerobic exercise; fat can *only* fuel aerobic activity. Our goal should be not to lose *weight* (although we most likely will lose weight as we increase our fitness levels), but to lose *fat*. To burn fat, *aerobic* activity is required, and that requires low to moderate intensity exercise. If the exercise is not intense enough, you will not burn sufficient calories to effect significant loss of fat; if it is too intense, two things will happen: your body will switch from *aerobic* to *anaerobic* metabolism and you will no longer be able to use fat as fuel (since fat can only be burned with *aerobic* activity). This is why in order to lose fat, low – moderate intensity activity is better. Moderate-intensity physical activity means working hard enough to raise your heart rate into your target heart zone; you should break a sweat, yet not be so out of breath that you are unable to carry on a conversation (see the ACSM /AHA recommendations in Appendix 4). In summary then, you need *both* types of exercise for an effective fitness and weight control program: *aerobic* activity to improve cardiovascular fitness and *weight training* to build and preserve muscle mass. Finally, since muscle weighs more than fat and since your goal is *fat* loss and not necessarily *weight* loss, throw the scale away! You won't need it to see if you are becoming more fit; you'll know!

Less is More.

You would be surprised; maybe shocked if you knew how much food you usually eat each day. The average American needs 2000-2400 calories a day, but *consumes* approximately 3400 calories per day. Where do the extra calories go? They are stored as fat, of course, which is why adult and childhood obesity have reached epidemic proportions in the U.S. As Type 2 diabetes is linked to obesity, this devastating illness is increasing as well. You may wish to record everything you eat and drink during the course of a typical day. This will keep you accountable and help you to stay focused as you work toward your goals.

There is strong scientific evidence from animal studies that less caloric consumption leads to longevity. There is no need to "starve yourself," in fact, that is a poor way to lose weight since it lowers your metabolism and makes weight loss even more difficult. The key is portion control. If you prepare meals for yourself, you will be able to control portion sizes, but you may have a great deal of difficulty with this when dining out. Restaurants are notorious for huge portion sizes since they don't want patrons to go away hungry. If you eat out frequently, plan to bring home a "doggie bag."

Stay Knowledgeable.

It goes without saying that you are ultimately responsible for your own health. Not the doctors or the nurses or the government, but you! Be proactive. The secret to life is not having all the answers, but being able to ask the right questions. Do not be afraid to ask. Be confident and set realistic goals for yourself. Stay knowledgeable about where your health information comes from. If something sounds too good to be true, it probably is. Continue to stay informed. For example, a new risk factor for heart disease has recently been identified: a protein marker in the blood known as *c-reactive protein* and it indicates the presence of inflammation. You will remember that heart disease is largely an inflammatory process and c-reactive protein may be one more link in the chain leading to heart disease. It has been known for some time that periodontal (gum) disease increases blood levels of this protein; another reason to keep your teeth and gums clean and healthy and get regular dental checkups. Other inflammatory conditions throughout the body may also contribute to it, so if your health care provider does not bring it up, then you mention it and ask to have it checked.

Play Your Hand Well!

To each is given a book of rules,
A shapeless mass and a bag of tools
And each must make 'ere life has flown
A stumbling block or a stepping stone.

–Author Unknown

If knowledge is power, you are now much stronger than you were before. You now know the difference between good fats and bad fats; you know the difference between good carbs and bad carbs. You know the importance of high quality protein; you know that water is essential for health. You know why it is so important to start your day with a healthy, nutritious breakfast. You know several important vitamins, minerals, and herbs and the role each plays in promoting and maintaining health. You know how to rate and compare the nutritional qualities of virtually any food. You now have the tools needed to play whatever hand you've been dealt. Play it well, my friend, play it well!

REFERENCES

Chapter 1: All Fats Are Not Bad

1. Mokdad AH, Serdula MK, Dietz WH, Bowman BA, Marks JS, & Koplan JP. The spread of the obesity epidemic in the United States, 1991-1998. *JAMA*. 1999; 282:1519.

2. Cholesterol levels, American Heart Association website, retrieved on 10/27/08 from http://www.americanheart.org/presenter.jhtml?identifier =4500heart.org.

3. McMichael AJ, Potter JD. Host factors in carcinogenesis: certain bile acid metabolic profiles that selectively increase the risk of proximal colon cancer. *J Natl Cancer Inst*.1985; 75:185-191.

4. DeRubertis FR, Craven PA. Relationship of bile salt stimulation of colonic epithelial phospholipid turnover and proliferative activity: role of activation of protein kinase *C.Prev Me.d*.1987; 16:572- 579.

5. Adlercreutz H. Diet, breast cancer and sex hormone metabolism. *Ann NY Acad Sci*.1990; 595: 281-290.

6. Holmes, Michelle D. Association of Dietary Intake of fat and fatty acids with risk of breast cancer. *JAMA*.1999 Mar; 28:10.

7. Summary of the Second Report of the National Cholesterol Education Program (NCEP) Expert Panel on Detection, Evaluation, and Treatment of High Blood Cholesterol in Adults (Adult Treat-ment Panel). *JAMA*.1993;269:3015-23.

8. Parkinson AJ, Cruz AL, Heyward WL, Bulkow LR, Hall D, Barstaed L, Connor WE. Elevated concentration of plasma omega-3 polyunsaturated fatty acids among Alaskan Eskimos. *Am J Clin Nutr*. 1994;59:384-388.

9. Lancet. 1994 (June 11);343:1454-9.

10. Flickinger BD, Huth PJ. Dietary fats and oils; technologies for improving cardiovascular health. *Curr Atheroscler Rep. 2004*;6:468-476.

11. Calder PC. n-3 fatty acids and cardiovascular disease: evidence explained and mechanisms explored. *Clin Sci (Lond)*. 2004;107:1-11.

12. Renaud SC. Diet and stroke. *J nutr Health Aging*. 2001;5:167-172.

13. Gerber MJ, Scali JD, Michaud A, et al. Profiles of a healthful diet and its relationship to biomarkers in a population sample from mediterranean southern France. *J Am Diet Assoc*.2000;100:1164-1171.

14. Simopoulos AP. Omega-3 fatty acids in inflammation and autoimmune diseases. *J Am Coll Nutr*. 2002;21:495-505.

PLAY YOUR HAND WELL

15. Uauy R, Foffman DR, Peirano P, et al. Essential fatty acids in visual and brain development. *Lipids*. 2001;36:885-895.

16. Belluzzi A, Boschi S, Brignola C, et al. Polyunsaturated fatty acids and inflammatory bowel disease. *Am J Clin Nutr*. 2000;71S:339S-342S.

17. Rose DP. Effects of dietary fatty acids on breast and prostate cancers: evidence from in vitro experiments and animal studies. *Am J Clin Nutr*. 1997;66S:1513S-1522S.

18. de Deckere EA. Possible beneficial effect of fish and fish n-3 polyunsaturated fatty acids in breast and colorectal cancer. *Eur J Cancer Prev*. 1999;8:213-221.

19. LaRosa, John C. Easy to digest answers to your patients' questions about diet and cholesterol. *Modern Medicine* 1994 Jun;62:36.

20. Willett WC, Stampfer MJ, Manson JE, et al. Intake of trans fatty acids and risk of coronary heart disease among women. *Lancet* 1993;341:581-5.

21. Mensink RP, Katan MB. Effect of dietary trans fatty acids on high-density and low-density lipoprotein levels in healthy subjects. *N Engl J Med* 1990;323:439-45.

22. Asherio A, Katan MB, Zock PL, Stampfer MJ, Willett WC. Trans fatty acids and coronary heart disease. *N Engl J Med*. 1999;340:1994-1998.

1. Jenkins, David J.A., et al. Glycemic index of foods: a physiological basis for carbohydrate exchange. *American Journal of Clinical Nutrition* 1981 Mar;34:362- 366.

2. Trout D., et al. Prediction of glycemic index among high-sugar, low-starch foods. *Int J Food Sci Nutr.* 1999 Mar;50:135-44.

3. Morris K.L., et al. Glycemic index, cardiovascular disease, and obesity. *Nutr Rev.* 1999 Sep;57:237-6.

4. Hellmich, N. Families ease heavy burden by shaping healthy habits. *USA Today* 1999 Aug 31.

5. Howe GR, Benito E, Castelleto R, Cornee J, Esteve J, Gallagher RP, Iscovich JM, Deng-ao J, Kaaks-Kune GA. Dietary intake of fiber and decreased risk of cancers of the colon and rectum: evidence from the combined analysis of 13 case-control studies. *J Natl Cancer Inst.* 1992;84: 1887-1896.

6. Wolever T.M.S., Jenkins D.J.A. Effect of dietary fiber and foods on carbohydrate metabolism. In: Spiller GA, ed. *CRC Handbook of Dietary Fiber in Human Nutrition.* 2nd ed. Boca Raton, Fla: CRC Press;1993:111-152.

7. Food and Nutrition Board, Institute of Medicine, Panel on the Definition of Dietary Fiber, Standing Committee on the Scientific Evaluation of Reference Intakes. Dietary Reference Intakes: Proposed Definition of Dietary Fiber. Washington, DC: National Academies Press; 2001. Available online at: http://darwin.nap.edu/books/0309075645/html.

8. Lampe, Johanna W. Health effects of vegetables and fruits: assessing mechanisms of action in human experimental studies. *Am J Clin Nutr* 1999;70:475-490.

9. Reddy ST, Wang CY, Sakhaee K, et al. Effect of low-carbohydrate high-protein diets on acid-base balance, stone-forming propensity, and calcium metabolism. *Am J Kidney Dis.* 2002;40:265-274.

10. Freedman MR, King J, Kennedy E. Popular diets: a scientific review. *Obes Res.* 2001;9:1S-40S.

Chapter 3: If Some Protein is Good, Is More Better?

1. *New England Journal of Medicine* 1994 (June 23);330:1776-1781.

2. Allen LH, Oddoye EA, Margen S. Protein-induced hypercalciuria: a longer term study. *Am J Clin Nutr* 1979;32: 741-749.

3. Anand JB, Linkswiler HM. Effect of protein intake on calcium balance of young men given 500 mg calcium daily. *J Nutr* 1974; 104:695-700.

4. Messina MJ. Legumes and soybeans: overview of their nutritional profiles and health effects. *Am J Clin Nutr* 1999;70:439-450.

5. Mix JA. Do megadoses of vitamin C compromise folic acid's role in the metabolism of plasma homocysteine? *Nutrition Research* 1999;19(2):161-165.

Chapter 4: Breakfast is Good

1. Kushi L.H., Lenart E.B., & Willett W.C. Health implications of Mediterranean diet in light of contemporary knowledge. *Am J Clin Nutr* 1995;61:1416S-1427S.

Chapter 5: Water is Good

1. Ziegler E.E., Filer L.J., eds. "Present Knowledge in Nutrition" 7th ed., International Life Sciences Institute. ILSI Press, Washington D.C, 1996, p. 107.

2. Rehrer N, Burke L. Sweat losses during various sports. *Aust J Nutr Diet* 1996;53:S13-16.

3. Weaver CM, Proulx Wr, Heaney RP. Choices for achieving dietary calcium within a vegetarian diet. *Am J Clin Nutr.* 1999;70:543S-548S

Chapter 6: Some Vitamin Supplements are Good

1. Cooper KH. "Antioxidant Revolution," Thomas Nelson Publishers, Nashville, 1994, p.12.

2. Linus Pauling biography, Linus Pauling Institute, Oregon State University website, retrieved on 11/5/08 from http://lpi.oregonstate.edu/lpbio/lpbio2.html.

3. Pawlak L. "A Perfect 10: Phyto 'New-trients' Against Cancers," Biomed General Corp.,Emeryville,CA, 1998,p.121.

4. Douglas RM, Hernila H, D'Souza R, Chalker EB, Treacy B. Vitamin C for preventing and treating the common cold. *Cochrane Database Syst R ev.* 2004(4): CD000980. (PubMed).

5. Enstrom JE, Kanim LE, Klein MA. Vitamin C intake and mortality among a sample of the United States population. *Epidemiology* 1992;3(3):194-202.

6. Micronutrient Information Center, Linus Pauling Institute, Oregon State University website, retrieved on 11/5/08 from http://lpi.oregonstate.edu/infocenter/vitamins/vitaminC/.

7. Solomons NW. "Vitamin A" in *Present Knowledge in Nutrition*, 9th ed.,vol.1, ILSI Press, Washington D.C., 2006, p.157-183.

8. Goodman GE, Thornquist MD, Balmes J, et al. The Beta-Carotene and Retinol Efficacy Trial: incidence of lung cancer and cardiovascular disease mortality during 6-year follow-up after stopping beta-carotene and retinol supplenments. *J Natl Cancer Inst.* 2004;96:1743-1750.

9. Vivekananthan DP, Penn MS, Sapp SK Hsu A, Topol EJ. Use of antioxidant vitamins for the prevention of cardiovascular disases: meta-analysis of randomized trials. *Lancet.*2003;361: 2017-2023.

10. Cooper KH. "Antioxidant Revolution," Thomas Nelson Publishers, Nashville, 1994, p.146.

11. Lindshield, BL, Erdman, Jr.,JW. "Carotenoids" in *Present Knowledge in Nutrition*, 9th ed.,vol.1, ILSI Press, Washington D.C., 2006, p.190-193.

12. Evans HM, Bishop KS. On the existence of a hitherto unrecognized dietary factor essential for reproduction. *Science* 1922;56:650-651.

13. Ascherio A, Weisskopf MG, O'Reilly EJ, et al. Vitamin E intake and risk of amyotrophic lateral sclerosis. *Ann Neuro.*2005;57:104-110.

14. Sano M, Ernesto C, Thomas RG, et al. A controlled trial of selegiline, alpha-tocopherol, or both as treatment for Alzheimer's disease. The Alzheimer's Disease Cooperative Study. *N Engl J Med.* 1997;336:1216-1222.

15. Sokol R. "Vitamin E" in Present Knowledge in Nutrition, 7th ed., ILSI Press, Washington D.C.,1996, p.132-133.

16. Pawlak L. "A Perfect 10: Phyto 'New-trients' Against Cancers," Biomed General Corp., Emeryville, CA, 1998,p.82.

17. Cooper KH. "Antioxidant Revolution," Thomas Nelson Publishers, Nashville, 1994, p.123.

18. Norman AW, Henry HH. "Vitamin D" in Present Knowledge in Nutrition, 9th ed.,vol.1, ILSI Press, Washington D.C., 2006, p.203-204.

19. Wagner CL, Greer FR. Prevention of rickets and vitamin D deficiency in infants, children, and adolescents. *American Academy of Pediatrics.* 2008;122(5):1142-1152. Available online at: http://www.aap.org/new/VitaminDreport.pdf

PLAY YOUR HAND WELL

● ● ● ● ● ● ●

20. Food and Nutrition Board, Institute of Medicine, Dietary Reference Intakes: A risk assessment model for establishing upper intake levels for nutrients. Washington, DC: National Academies Press; 1998. Available at: http://nap.edu/openbook/0309063485/html.

21. Culbert ML. "Vitamin B17: Forbidden Weapon Against Cancer," Arlington House Publishers New Rochelle, NY, 1974, p. 93.

22. Mix JA. The effects of amygdalin on the S91 Melanoma in ICR mice. unpublished clinical research, senior thesis, Dickinson College, Carlisle, PA, 1975.

23. Carmel R, Gott PS, Waters CH, et al. The frequently low cobalamin levels in dementia usually signify treatable metabolic, neurologic and electrophysiologic abnormalities. *Eur J Haematol.* 1995;54:245-253.

Chapter 7: Some Mineral Supplements Are Good, Too!

1. Recker RR, Davies KM, Hinders SM, et al. Bone gain in young adult women. *JAMA* 1992;268:2403-2408.

2. Bonjour JP, Theintz G, Buchs B. Critical years and stages of puberty for spinal and femoral bone mass accumulation during adolescence. *J CLin Endocrinol Metab* 1991;73:555-563.

3. Goulding A, Rochell JP, Black RE, et al. Children who avoid drinking cow's milk are at increased risk for prepubertal bone fractures. *J Am Diet Assoc.* 2004;104:250-253.

4. Food and Nutrition Board, Institute of Medicine. Dietary Reference Intakes for Calcium, Phosphorus, Magnesium, Vitamin D, and Fluoride. Washington, DC: National Academies Press; 1997. Available online at: http://nap.edu/books/0309063507/html.

5. Lipkin M, Newmark H. Calcium and the prevention of colon cancer. *J Cell Biochem* 1995; 22(suppl):65-73.

6. Wu K, Wllett WC, Fuchs CS, Colditz GA, Giovanucchi EL. Calcium intake and risk of colon cancer in women and men. *J Natl Cancer Inst.* 2002;94:437-446.

7. Lamprecht SA, Lipkin M. Chemoprevention of colon cancer by calcium, vitamin D and folate: molecular mechanisms. *Nat Rev Cancer.* 2003;3:601-614.

8. Appel LJ, Moore TJ, Obarzanek E, et al. A clinical trial of the effects of dietary patterns of blood pressure. *N Engl J Med.* 1997;336:1117-1124.

9. Iso H, Stampfer MJ, Manson JE, et al. Prospective study of calcium, potassium, and magnesium intake and risk of stroke in women. *Stroke* 1999;30:1772-1779.

10. Curhan GC, Willett WC, Rumm EB, et al. A protective study of dietary calcium and other nutrients and the risk of symptomatic kidney stones. *N Engl J Med* 1993;328:833-838.

11. Thys-Jacobs S, Starhey P, Bernstein D, Tian J. Calcium carbonate and premenstrual syndrome: effects on premenstrual and menstrual symptoms. *Am J Obstet Gynecol* 1998;179:444-452.

12. Seppa N. Mediterranean diet proves value again. *Science News* 1999 Feb;155:119.

13. Ellenhorn MJ, Barceloux DG, eds. "Iron" in Medical Toxicology. *Elsevier*, New York, 1988 p. 1023-1030.

Chapter 8: Herbal Medicinals: The Good, The Bad, and the "We Don't Really Know"

1. Mix JA, Crews WD. A double-blind, placebo-controlled, randomized trial of *Ginkgo biloba* extract EGb 761® in a sample of cognitively intact older adults: neuropsychological findings. *Hum Psychopharmacol Clin Exp* 2002;17:267-277.

2. Mix JA, Crews WD. An examination of the efficacy of Ginkgo biloba extract EGb 761 on the neuropsychological functioning of cognitively intact older adults. *The Journal of Alternative and Complementary Medicine* 2000;6(3): p.219-229.

3. Gruenwald J, Brendler T, and Jaenicke C, eds. "PDR for Herbal Medicines," 4th edition, Thomson Healthcare, Montvale, NJ, 2007, p. 345-353.

4. Tyler VE. "Herbs of Choice: The Therapeutic Use of Phytomedicinals," Pharmaceutical Products Press, Binghamptom, NY, 1994. p. 105.

5. Lau BH. Suppression of LDL oxidation by garlic compounds is a possible mechanism of cardiovascular health benefit. *J Nutr* 2006; 36(3 Suppl):765S-768S.

6. Josling P. Preventing the common cold with a Garlic supplement: a double-blind, placebo-controlled survey. *Adv Ther* 2001;18(4):189-193.

7. Gruenwald J, Brendler T, and Jaenicke C, eds. "PDR for Herbal Medicines," 4th edition, Thomson Healthcare, Montvale, NJ, 2007, p. 579.

8. Zakay-Rones Z, Thom E, Wollan T, et al. Randomized study of the efficacy and safety of oral Elderberry extract in the treatment of influenza A and B virus infections .*J Int Med Res* 2004;32(2):132-140.

9. Tyler VE. "Herbs of Choice: The Therapeutic Use of Phytomedicinals," Pharmaceutical Products Press, Binghamptom, NY, 1994. p.163.

10. Tyler VE. "Herbs of Choice: The Therapeutic Use of Phytomedicinals," Pharmaceutical Products Products Press, Binghamptom, NY, 1994. p.163.

11. Gruenwald J, Brendler T, and Jaenicke C, eds. "PDR for Herbal Medicines," 4th edition, Thomson Healthcare, Montvale, NJ, 2007, p.596.

12. Ody P. "The Complete Medicinal Herbal," Dorling Kindersley Limited, London, 1993,p. 75.

13. Arjmandi BH, Khan DA, Juma S et al. Whole flaxseed consumption lower serum LDL cholesterol and lipoprotein(a) concentrations in postmenopausal women. In: *Nutr Res* 1998;18(7):1203-1214.

14. Nestle PJ, Pomeroy SE, Sasahara T et al. Arterial compliance in obese subjects is improved with dietary plant n-3 fatty acid from flaxseed oil despite increased LDL oxidizability. *Arterioscler Thromb Vasc Biol* 1997;17(6):1163-1170.

15. Thompson LU, Chen JM, Li T, et al. Dietary flaxseed alters tumor biological markers in post-menopausal breast cancer. *Clin Cancer Res* 2005; 11(10):3828-3835.

16. Gruenwald J, Brendler T, and Jaenicke C, eds. "PDR for Herbal Medicines," 4th edition, Thomson Healthcare, Montvale, NJ, 2007, p. 330.

17. Allman MA, Pena MM and Pang D. Supplementation with flaxseed oil versus sunflower seed oil in healthy young men consuming a low fat diet: effects on platelet composition and function. In: *Eur J Clin Nutr* 1995;49(3):169-178.

18. Gruenwald J, Brendler T, and Jaenicke C, eds. "PDR for Herbal Medicines," 4th edition, Thomson Healthcare, Montvale, NJ, 2007, p. 414.

19. Kannar ML, Wahlqvist ML and O'Brien RC. Inhibition of LDL oxidation by Green Tea extract. *Lancet* 1997;349:360-361.

20. Yamamoto T, Juneja LR, Chu DC et al., "Chemistry and Applications of Green Tea," CRC Press, Boca Raton, FL, USA,1997.

21. Aucamp J. Inhibition of xanthine oxidase by catechins from tea (Camellia sinesis). *Anticancer Res* 1997;17:4381-4386.

REFERENCES

● ● ● ● ● ● ●

22. Iso H, Date C, Kenji W, et al. The relationship between Green Tea and total caffeine intake and risk for self-reported type 2 diabetes among Japanese adults. *Ann Intern Med* 2006; 144(8):554-562.

23. Vutyavanich T, et al. Ginger for nausea and vomiting in pregnancy: randomized, double-masked, placebo-controlled trial. *Obstet Gynecol* 2001;97(4):577-582.

24. Srivastava KC and Mustafa T. Ginger (Zingiber officinale) in rheumatism and musculoskeletal disorders. *Med hypotheses* 1992;39(4):342-348.

25. Gruenwald J, Brendler T, and Jaenicke C, eds. "PDR for Herbal Medicines," 4th edition, Thomson Healthcare, Montvale, NJ, 2007, p.366.

26. Tyler VE. "Herbs of Choice: The Therapeutic Use of Phytomedicinals," Pharmaceutical Products Press, Binghamptom, NY, 1994. p. 82.

27. Wilt TJ, Ishani A, Rutks I et al. Phytotherapy for benign prostatic hyperplasia. *Public Health Nutr* 2000;2(4a):459-472.

28. Tyler VE. "Herbs of Choice: The Therapeutic Use of Phytomedicinals," Pharmaceutical Products Press, Binghamptom, NY, 1994. p.135.

29. Schellenberg R. Treatment for the premenstrual syndrome with agnus castus fruit extract: prospective, randomized, placeb controlled study. In: *BMJ* 2001;322(7279):134-147.

30. Prilepskaya V, Ledina AV, Tagiyeva AV, et al. Vitex agnus castus: successful treatment of moderate to severe premenstrual syndrome. In: *Maturitas* 2006;55S:S55-S63.

31. Gruenwald J, Brendler T, and Jaenicke C, eds. "PDR for Herbal Medicines," 4th edition, Thomson Healthcare, Montvale, NJ, 2007, p.268.

32. Vestweber AM, Beuth J, Ko HL et al. In vitro activity of Mercuris cyanatus complex against relevant pathogenic bacterial isolates (German). *Arzneimittelforschung* 1995; 45(9):1018-1020.

33. Goel V, Lovin R, Chang C, et al. A proprietary extract from the Echinacea plant (Echinacea purpurea) enhances systemic immune response during common cold. *Phytother Res* 2005; 19(8):689-694.

34. Goel V, Lovin R, Bartion R, et al. Efficacy of a standardized Echinacea preparation (Echinilin) for the treatment of the common cold: a randomized, double-blind, placeb-controlled trial. *J Clin Pharm Ther* 2004; 29(1):75-83.

35. Sperber SJ, Shah LP, Gilbert RD, et al. Echinacea purpurea for prevention of experimental rhinovirus colds. *Clin Infect Dis* 2004;38(10):1367-1371.

36. Lindenmuth GF and Lindenmuth EB. The efficacy of Echinacea compound herbal tea preparation on the severity and duration of upper respiratory and flu symptoms: a randomized, double-blind, placebo-controlled study. *J Alt Compl Med* 2000; 6(4):327-333.

37. Henneicke-von Sepelin HH, Hentschel C, Schnitker J et al. Efficacy and safety of a fixed combination phytomedicine in the treatment of the common cold (acute viral respiratory tract infection):result of a randomized, double-blind, placebo-controlled clinical trial. *Curr Med Res Op* 1999; 15(3):213-227.

38. Hoheisel O, Sandberg M, Bertram S et al. Echinagard treatment shortens the course of the common cold: a double-blind, placebo-controlled clinical trial. *Eur J Clin Res* 1997; 9:261-268.

39. Schultz V and Haensel R. Rationale Phytotherapie (German). Ratgeber fuer die aertzlich Praxis. 3 Aufl. Springer Verlag, Berlin, Germany 1996.

Chapter 9: The Mix Food Quality Index™ and the Top 10 Foods

1. USDA Nutrient Data Laboratory, USDA National Nutrient Database for Standard Reference at: http://www.nal.usda.gov/fnic/foodcomp/search/

2. Food and Nutrition Board, Institute of Medicine, Dietary Reference Intakes for Vitamin C, Vitamin E, Selenium, and Carotenoids. Washington, DC: National Academies Press; 2000. Available online at: http://nap.edu/openbook/0309069351/html/index.html.

3. Cooper KH. "Antioxidant Revolution," Thomas Nelson Publishers, Nashville, 1994, p.146.

4. WHO Technical Report Series."Diet, Nutrition, and the Prevention of Chronic Diseases" Report of a Joint FAO/WHO Consultation. Geneva. 2003.p.56. Available online at: http://whqlibdoc.who.int/trs/WHO_TRS_916.pdf. Accessed November 19, 2008.

5. Boutrif E. Food Quality and Consumer Protection Group, Food Policy and Nutrition Division, FAO, Rome: "Recent Developments in Protein Quality Evaluation," *Food, Nutrition and Agriculture*, 1991;2/3.

6. Adapted from: Sizer F, Whitney E. "Nutrition Concepts and Controversies," 8th edition, Wadsworth Thomson Learning, Belmont, CA, 2000.p.190-194.

7. Pawlak L. "A Perfect 10: Phyto 'New-trients' Against Cancers," Biomed General Corp., Emeryville, CA, 1998,p.113.

APPENDICES

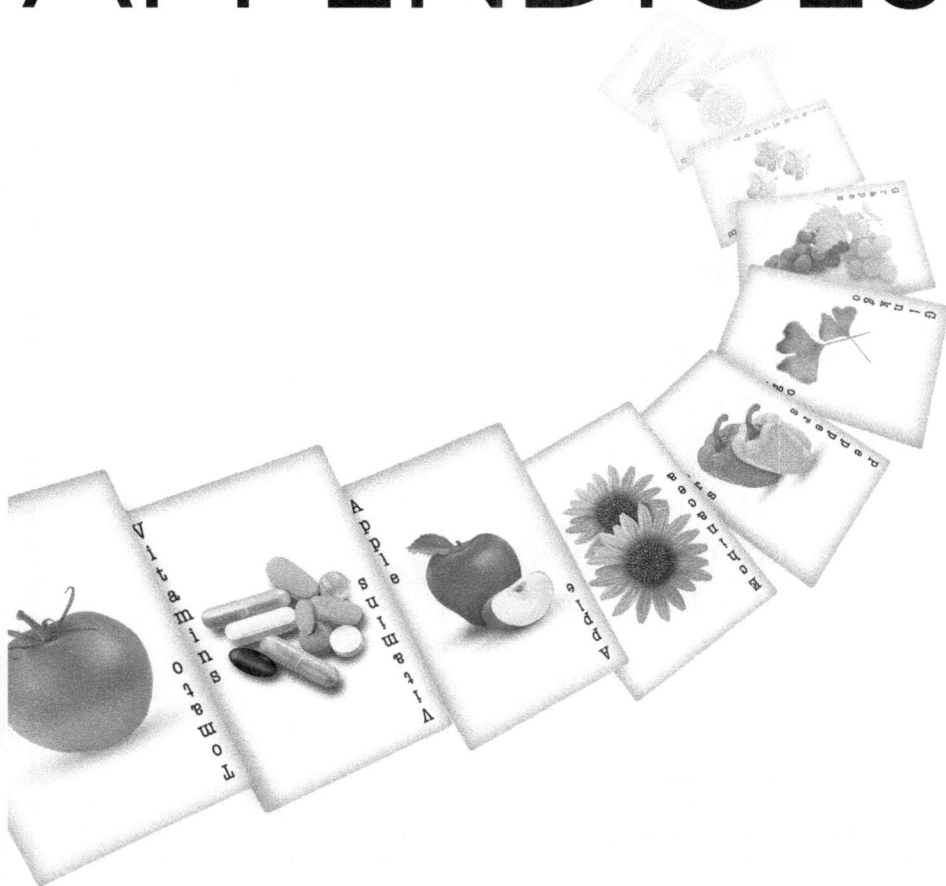

APPENDIX 1A. The Mix Food Quality Index ™ Score for Selected Foods.

INDEX	NUTRIENT	RA[1]	UNIT	CARROT (488 grams/200 kcal)[2]		
				Amt.	% RA	Score
A P I	Vitamin C	90	mg	28.8	32.0	1
	Beta-carotene	15	mg	40.4	269.5	1
	Vitamin E	15	mg	3.2	21.5	1
	Selenium	55	mcg	0.5	0.9	0.09
	TOTAL (API)					**3.09**
C S I	Calcium	1000	mg	161.0	16.1	1
	Potassium	4700	mg	1562.0	33.2	1
	Magnesium	370	mg	59.0	15.9	1
	MUFA[3]	15	g	0.1	0.7	0.07
	Omega-3[4]	4	g	0	0	0
	Fiber[5]	26	g	13.7	52.7	1
	TOTAL (CSI)					**4.07**
P D I	Protein (Quantity)[6]	75	g	4.5	6.0	0.60
	Protein (Quality)[7]					0.20
	TOTAL (PDI)					**0.80**
N I H	SAT FAT[8]	22	g	0.2	0.9	0.09
	TRANS FAT[9]	2	g	0	0	0
	Sugars[10]	50	g	23.1	46.2	1
	Sodium	1500	mg	337.0	22.4	1
	TOTAL (NIH)					**2.09**
MIX FOOD QUALITY INDEX (API + CSI + PDI) – NIH						**5.87**

PEANUT (35 grams/200 kcal)[2]			BROCCOLI (588 grams/200 kcal)[2]		
Amt.	% RA	Score	Amt.	% RA	Score
0	0	0	524.5	582.7	1
0	0	0	2.1	14.1	1
2.94	19.6	1	4.6	30.6	1
2.5	4.5	0.45	14.7	26.7	1
		1.45			**4.00**
32.0	3.2	0.32	276.0	27.6	1
249.0	5.3	0.53	1858.0	39.5	1
59.00	15.9	1	123.0	33.2	1
8.6	57.3	1	0.1	0.6	0.06
0	0	0	0.1	2.5	0.25
3.0	11.5	1	15.3	58.8	1
		3.85			**4.31**
9.1	12.1	1	16.6	22.1	1
		0.50			0.30
		1.50			**1.30**
2.4	10.9	1	0.2	0.9	0.09
0	0	0	0	0	0
1.4	2.8	0.28	10.0	20.0	1
6.0	0.4	0.04	194.0	12.9	1
		1.32			**2.09**
		5.48			**7.52**

INDEX	NUTRIENT	RA[1]	UNIT	RED PEPPER (645 grams/200kcal)[2]		
				Amt.	% RA	Score
A P I	Vitamin C	90	mg	823.7	915.2	1
	Beta-carotene	15	mg	10.5	70.0	1
	Vitamin E	15	mg	10.2	68.0	1
	Selenium	55	mcg	0.6	1.1	0.11
	TOTAL (API)					**3.11**
C S I	Calcium	1000	mg	45.0	4.5	0.45
	Potassium	4700	mg	1361.0	28.9	1
	Magnesium	370	mg	77.0	20.8	1
	MUFA[3]	15	g	0	0	0
	Omega-3[4]	4	g	0	0	0
	Fiber[5]	26	g	13.5	51.9	1
	TOTAL (CSI)					**3.45**
P D I	Protein (Quantity)[6]	75	g	6.4	8.5	0.85
	Protein (Quality)[7]					0.20
	TOTAL (PDI)					**1.05**
N I H	SAT FAT[8]	22	g	0.2	0.9	0.09
	TRANS FAT[9]	2	g	0	0	0
	Sugars[10]	50	g	27.1	54.2	1
	Sodium	1500	mg	26.0	1.7	0.17
	TOTAL (NIH)					**1.26**
MIX FOOD QUALITY INDEX (API + CSI + PDI) – NIH						**6.35**

SWEET POTATO (233 grams/200kcal)[2]			GRAPE (290 grams/200kcal)[2]		
Amt.	% RA	Score	Amt.	% RA	Score
5.6	6.2	0.62	31.3	34.7	1
19.8	132.0	1	0.1	0.7	0.07
0.6	4.0	0.40	0.55	3.7	0.37
1.4	2.5	0.25	0.3	0.5	0.05
		2.27			**1.49**
70.0	7.0	0.70	29	2.9	0.29
785.0	16.7	1	554.0	11.8	1
58.0	15.7	1	20.0	5.4	0.54
0	0	0	0	0	0
0	0	0	0	0	0
7.0	26.9	1	2.6	10.0	1
		3.70			**2.83**
3.66	4.8	0.48	2.09	2.8	0.28
		0.20			0.10
		0.68			**0.38**
0	0	0	0.2	0.9	0.09
0	0	0	0	0	0
9.7	19.4	1	44.9	89.8	1
128.0	8.5	0.85	6.0	0.4	0.04
		1.85			**1.13**
		4.80			**3.57**

INDEX	NUTRIENT	RA[1]	UNIT	ONION (500 grams/200kcal)[2]		
				Amt.	% RA	Score
A P I	Vitamin C	90	mg	37.0	41.1	1
	Beta-carotene	15	mg	0	0	0
	Vitamin E	15	mg	0.1	0.7	0.07
	Selenium	55	mcg	2.5	4.5	0.45
	TOTAL (API)					1.52
C S I	Calcium	1000	mg	115.0	11.5	1
	Potassium	4700	mg	730.0	15.5	1
	Magnesium	370	mg	50.0	13.5	1
	MUFA[3]	15	g	0.1	0.7	0.07
	Omega-3[4]	4	g	0	0	0
	Fiber[5]	26	g	8.5	32.7	1
	TOTAL (CSI)					4.07
P D I	Protein (Quantity)[6]	75	g	5.5	7.3	0.73
	Protein (Quality)[7]					0.20
	TOTAL (PDI)					0.93
N I H	SAT FAT[8]	22	g	0.2	0.9	0.09
	TRANS FAT[9]	2	g	0	0	0
	Sugars[10]	50	g	21.2	42.4	1
	Sodium	1500	mg	20.0	1.3	0.13
	TOTAL (NIH)					1.22
MIX FOOD QUALITY INDEX (API + CSI + PDI) – NIH						5.30

WHEAT GERM (56 grams/200kcal)^2			SOYBEAN (44.9 grams/200kcal)^2		
Amt.	% RA	Score	Amt.	% RA	Score
0	0	0	2.7	3.0	0.30
0	0	0	0	0	0
9.4	62.7	1	0.4	2.7	0.27
44.0	80.0	1	8.0	14.5	1
		2.00			**1.57**
22.0	2.2	0.20	124.0	12.4	1
495.0	10.5	1	807.0	17.2	1
133.0	35.9	1	126.0	34.1	1
0.8	5.3	0.53	2.0	13.3	1
0.4	10.0	1	0.6	15.0	1
7.3	28.1	1	4.2	16.2	1
		4.73			**6.00**
12.9	17.2	1	16.4	21.9	1
		0.40			0.90
		1.40			**1.90**
0.9	4.1	0.41	1.3	5.9	0.59
0	0	0	0	0	0
0	0	0	3.29	6.6	0.66
7.0	0.5	0.05	1.0	0.1	0.01
		0.46			**1.26**
		7.67			**8.21**

APPENDIX 1D. The Mix Food Quality Index ™ Score for Selected Foods.

INDEX	NUTRIENT	RA[1]	UNIT	TOMATO (1112 grams/200kcal)[2]		
				Amt.	% RA	Score
A P I	Vitamin C	90	mg	141.2	156.9	1
	Beta-carotene	15	mg	5.0	33.3	1
	Vitamin E	15	mg	6.0	40.0	1
	Selenium	55	mcg	0	0	0
	TOTAL (API)					**3.00**
C S I	Calcium	1000	mg	111.0	11.1	1
	Potassium	4700	mg	2635.0	56.1	1
	Magnesium	370	mg	122.0	32.9	1
	MUFA[3]	15	g	0.3	2.0	0.20
	Omega-3[4]	4	g	0	0	0
	Fiber[5]	26	g	13.3	51.2	1
	TOTAL (CSI)					**4.20**
P D I	Protein (Quantity)[6]	75	g	9.8	13.1	1
	Protein (Quality)[7]					0.20
	TOTAL (PDI)					**1.20**
N I H	SAT FAT[8]	22	g	0.3	1.4	0.14
	TRANS FAT[9]	2	g	0	0	0
	Sugars[10]	50	g	29.3	58.5	1
	Sodium	1500	mg	56.0	3.7	0.37
	TOTAL (NIH)					**1.51**
MIX FOOD QUALITY INDEX (API + CSI + PDI) – NIH						**6.89**

CANDY (M&M's) (41 grams/200kcal)[2]			HOT DOG (60.6 grams/200kcal)[2]		
Amt.	% RA	Score	Amt.	% RA	Score
0	0	0	0	0	0
0	0	0	0	0	0
0.2	1.0	0.10	0.1	0.7	0.07
1.3	2.4	0.24	5	9.1	0.91
		0.34			**0.98**
43.0	4.3	0.43	8.0	0.8	0.08
106.0	2.2	0.22	95.0	2.0	0.20
18.0	4.9	0.49	8.0	2.2	0.22
2.1	14.0	1	8.7	58.0	1
0	0	0	0.1	2.5	0.25
1.1	4.2	0.42	0	0	0
		2.56			**1.75**
1.76	2.3	0.23	6.81	9.1	0.91
		0			1
		0.23			**1.91**
5.3	24.1	1	7.1	32.3	1
0.1	5.0	0.50	0	0	0
25.9	51.8	1	2.1	4.2	0.42
25.0	1.7	0.17	691.0	46.1	1
		2.67			**2.42**
		0.46			**2.22**

APPENDIX 1E. The Mix Food Quality Index ™ Score for Selected Foods.

INDEX	NUTRIENT	RA[1]	UNIT	CHICKEN (with skin) (116 grams/200kcal)[2]		
				Amt.	% RA	Score
A P I	Vitamin C	90	mg	0	0	0
	Beta-carotene	15	mg	0	0	0
	Vitamin E	15	mg	0.4	2.7	0.27
	Selenium	55	mcg	19.3	35.1	1
	TOTAL (API)					**1.27**
C S I	Calcium	1000	mg	13.0	1.3	0.13
	Potassium	4700	mg	256.0	5.4	0.54
	Magnesium	370	mg	29.0	7.8	0.78
	MUFA[3]	15	g	4.5	30.0	1
	Omega-3[4]	4	g	0.1	2.5	0.25
	Fiber[5]	26	g	0	0	0
	TOTAL (CSI)					**2.70**
P D I	Protein (Quantity)[6]	75	g	24.29	32.4	1
	Protein (Quality)[7]					1
	TOTAL (PDI)					**2.00**
N I H	SAT FAT[8]	22	g	3.1	14.1	1
	TRANS FAT[9]	2	g	0	0	0
	Sugars[10]	50	g	0	0	0
	Sodium	1500	mg	73.0	4.9	0.49
	TOTAL (NIH)					**1.49**
MIX FOOD QUALITY INDEX (API + CSI + PDI) – NIH						**4.48**

CHICKEN (without skin) (182 grams/200kcal)[2]			FISH (Pink Salmon) (172 grams/200kcal)[2]		
Amt.	% RA	Score	Amt.	% RA	Score
0	0	0	0	0	0
0	0	0	0	0	0
0.2	1.3	0.13	1.1	7.3	0.73
32.4	58.9	1	76.7	139.4	1
		1.13			**1.73**
20.0	2.0	0.20	22.0	2.2	0.22
464.0	9.9	0.99	556.0	11.8	1
51.0	13.8	1	45.0	12.2	1
0.5	3.3	0.33	1.6	10.7	1
0.1	2.5	0.25	2.0	50.0	1
0	0	0	0	0	0
		2.77			**4.22**
42.02	56.0	1	34.30	45.7	1
		1			1
		2.00			**2.00**
0.6	2.7	0.27	1.0	4.5	0.45
0	0	0	0	0	0
0	0	0	0	0	0
118.0	7.9	0.79	115.0	7.7	0.77
		1.06			**1.22**
		4.84			**6.73**

APPENDIX 1F. The Mix Food Quality Index ™ Score for Selected Foods.

INDEX	NUTRIENT	RA[1]	UNIT	SPINACH (868 grams/200kcal)[2]		
				Amt.	% RA	Score
A P I	Vitamin C	90	mg	243.9	271.0	1
	Beta-carotene	15	mg	48.8	325.3	1
	Vitamin E	15	mg	17.6	117.3	1
	Selenium	55	mcg	8.7	15.8	1
	TOTAL (API)					**4.00**
C S I	Calcium	1000	mg	859.0	85.9	1
	Potassium	4700	mg	4843.0	103.0	1
	Magnesium	370	mg	686.0	185.4	1
	MUFA[3]	15	g	0.1	0.7	0.07
	Omega-3[4]	4	g	1.2	30.0	1
	Fiber[5]	26	g	19.1	73.4	1
	TOTAL (CSI)					**5.07**
P D I	Protein (Quantity)[6]	75	g	24.82	33.1	1
	Protein (Quality)[7]					0.30
	TOTAL (PDI)					**1.30**
N I H	SAT FAT[8]	22	g	0.5	2.3	0.23
	TRANS FAT[9]	2	g	0	0	0
	Sugars[10]	50	g	3.7	7.4	0.74
	Sodium	1500	mg	686.0	45.7	1
	TOTAL (NIH)					**1.97**
MIX FOOD QUALITY INDEX (API + CSI + PDI) − NIH						**8.40**

172

ALMOND (35 grams/200kcal)[2]			WHITE POTATO (290 grams/200kcal)[2]		
Amt.	% RA	Score	Amt.	% RA	Score
0	0	0	57.1	63.4	1
0	0	0	0	0	0
9.1	16.5	1	0	0	0
0.9	1.6	0.16	0.9	1.6	0.16
		1.16			**1.16**
92.0	9.2	0.92	26.0	2.6	0.26
245.0	5.2	0.52	1180.0	25.1	1
93.0	25.1	1	61.0	16.4	1
10.7	71.3	1	0	0	0
0	0	0	0	0	0
4.2	16.1	1	7.0	26.9	1
		4.44			**3.26**
7.36	9.8	0.98	4.87	6.6	0.65
		0.40			0.20
		1.38			**0.85**
1.3	5.9	0.59	0.1	0	0
0	0	0	0	0	0
1.4	2.8	0.28	3.3	6.6	0.66
0	0	0	17.0	1.1	0.11
		0.87			**0.77**
		6.11			**4.50**

APPENDIX 1G. The Mix Food Quality Index ™ Score for Selected Foods.

INDEX	NUTRIENT	RA[1]	UNIT	ORANGE (426 grams/200kcal)[2]		
				Amt.	% RA	Score
A P I	Vitamin C	90	mg	226.6	251.7	1
	Beta-carotene	15	mg	0.3	2.0	0.20
	Vitamin E	15	mg	0.8	5.3	0.53
	Selenium	55	mcg	2.1	3.8	0.38
	TOTAL (API)					**2.11**
C S I	Calcium	1000	mg	170.0	17.0	1
	Potassium	4700	mg	771.0	16.4	1
	Magnesium	370	mg	43.0	11.6	1
	MUFA[3]	15	g	0.1	0.7	0.07
	Omega-3[4]	4	g	0	0	0
	Fiber[5]	26	g	10.2	39.2	1
	TOTAL (CSI)					**4.07**
P D I	Protein (Quantity)[6]	75	g	4.0	5.3	0.53
	Protein (Quality)[7]					0.10
	TOTAL (PDI)					**0.63**
N I H	SAT FAT[8]	22	g	0	0	0
	TRANS FAT[9]	2	g	0	0	0
	Sugars[10]	50	g	39.8	79.6	1
	Sodium	1500	mg	0	0	0
	TOTAL (NIH)					**1.00**
MIX FOOD QUALITY INDEX (API + CSI + PDI) − NIH						**5.81**

CORN (233 grams/200kcal)²			FLAXSEED (37.4 grams/200kcal)²		
Amt.	% RA	Score	Amt.	% RA	Score
15.8	17.5	1	0.2	0.2	0.02
0.1	0.7	0.07	0	0	0
0.2	1.3	0.13	0.1	0.8	0.08
1.4	2.5	0.25	9.5	17.2	1
		1.45			**1.10**
5	0.5	0.05	95.0	9.5	0.95
629	13.4	1	304.0	6.4	0.64
86	23.2	1	147.0	39.7	1
0.8	5.3	0.53	2.8	18.7	1
0	0	0	8.5	212.5	1
6.3	24.2	1	10.2	39.2	1
		3.58			**5.59**
7.5	10.0	1	6.8	9.1	0.91
		0.40			0.40
		1.40			**1.31**
0.4	1.8	0.18	1.4	6.3	0.63
0	0	0	0	0	0
7.5	15.0	1	0.6	1.2	0.12
35.0	2.3	0.23	11.0	0.7	0.07
		1.41			**0.82**
		5.02			**7.18**

INDEX	NUTRIENT	RA[1]	UNIT	EGG (140 grams/200kcal)[2]		
				Amt.	% RA	Score
A P I	Vitamin C	90	mg	0.2	0.2	0.02
	Beta-carotene	15	mg	0	0	0
	Vitamin E	15	mg	1.4	9.1	0.91
	Selenium	55	mcg	44.3	80.5	1
	TOTAL (API)					1.93
C S I	Calcium	1000	mg	74.0	7.4	0.74
	Potassium	4700	mg	187.0	3.9	0.39
	Magnesium	370	mg	17.0	4.6	0.46
	MUFA[3]	15	g	5.3	35.3	1
	Omega-3[4]	4	g	0.1	2.5	0.25
	Fiber[5]	26	g	0	0	0
	TOTAL (CSI)					2.84
P D I	Protein (Quantity)[6]	75	g	17.6	23.4	1
	Protein (Quality)[7]					1
	TOTAL (PDI)					2.00
N I H	SAT FAT[8]	22	g	4.3	19.5	1
	TRANS FAT[9]	2	g	0	0	0
	Sugars[10]	50	g	1.1	2.2	0.22
	Sodium	1500	mg	196.0	13.1	1
	TOTAL (NIH)					2.22
MIX FOOD QUALITY INDEX (API + CSI + PDI) – NIH						4.55

HAMBURGER (79 grams/200kcal)[2]			FRENCH FRIES (68 grams/200kcal)[2]		
Amt.	% RA	Score	Amt.	% RA	Score
0	0	0	4.6	5.1	0.51
0	0	0	0	0	0
0.3	2.0	0.20	0	0	0
11.8	21.4	1	0	0	0
		1.20			0.51
14.0	1.4	0.14	11.0	1.1	0.11
213.0	4.5	0.45	354.0	7.5	0.75
13.0	3.5	0.35	20.0	5.4	0.54
6.9	46.0	1	4.9	32.7	1
0.1	2.5	0.25	0.2	5.0	0.05
0	0	0	2.7	10.4	1
		2.19			3.45
13.5	18.0	1	2.4	3.2	0.32
		1			0
		2.00			0.32
6.0	27.2	1	1.3	5.9	0.59
1.0	50.0	1	0.1	5.0	0.50
0	0	0	0.1	0.2	0.02
53.0	3.5	0.35	144.0	9.6	0.96
		2.35			2.07
		3.04			2.21

APPENDIX 1I. The Mix Food Quality Index ™ Score for Selected Foods.

INDEX	NUTRIENT	RA[1]	UNIT	CABBAGE (800 grams/200kcal)[2]		
				Amt.	% RA	Score
A P I	Vitamin C	90	mg	292.8	325.3	1
	Beta-carotene	15	mg	0.3	2.0	0.20
	Vitamin E	15	mg	1.2	8.0	0.80
	Selenium	55	mcg	2.4	4.4	0.44
	TOTAL (API)					**2.44**
C S I	Calcium	1000	mg	320.0	32.0	1
	Potassium	4700	mg	1360.0	28.9	1
	Magnesium	370	mg	96.0	25.9	1
	MUFA[3]	15	g	0.1	0.6	0.06
	Omega-3[4]	4	g	0	0	0
	Fiber[5]	26	g	20.0	76.9	1
	TOTAL (CSI)					**4.06**
P D I	Protein (Quantity)[6]	75	g	10.2	13.6	1
	Protein (Quality)[7]					0.30
	TOTAL (PDI)					**1.30**
N I H	SAT FAT[8]	22	g	0.3	1.4	0.14
	TRANS FAT[9]	2	g	0	0	0
	Sugars[10]	50	g	25.6	51.2	1
	Sodium	1500	mg	144.0	9.6	0.96
	TOTAL (NIH)					**2.10**
MIX FOOD QUALITY INDEX (API + CSI + PDI) – NIH						**5.70**

APPLE (384 grams/200kcal)[2]			YOUR FOOD HERE		
Amt.	% RA	Score	Amt.	% RA	Score
17.7	19.7	1			
0.1	0.7	0.07			
0.7	4.7	0.47			
0	0	0			
		1.54			
23.0	2.3	0.23			
411.0	8.7	0.87			
19.0	5.1	0.51			
0	0	0			
0	0	0			
9.2	35.4	1			
		2.61			
1.0	1.3	0.13			
		0.10			
		0.23			
0.1	0.5	0.05			
0	0	0			
39.9	79.8	1			
4.0	0.3	0.03			
		1.08			
		3.30			

APPENDIX 1A - 1I. Reference Numbers.

1. Recommended adult daily intake as established by a recognized authority such as the Institute of Medicine or the World Health Organization (WHO). In cases where there are different recommendations for males and females, the two have been averaged together for the purpose of facilitating scoring. There is no RDA for beta-carotene; the recommendation of 15 mg per day is based on Dr. Kenneth Cooper's recommendation of 15 mg beta-carotene per day from *food* only (see references).

2. The scoring system is based on the quantity of food required to yield 200 calories (1/10th of a daily calorie intake of 2000).

3. Monounsaturated fatty acids.

4. Omega-3 fatty acids.

5. Based on a 2000 calorie/day diet and the WHO recommendation of 10 – 13 grams per 1000 calories.

6. Based on the WHO recommendation of 10 – 15% of daily calories for a 2000 calorie per day diet.

7. As assessed by *estimates* of the PDCAAS (Protein Digestibility Corrected Amino Acid Score). See Table13.

8. Saturated Fat.

9. Trans Fat.

10. Based on the WHO recommendation of no more than 10% of calories per day from sugar for a 2000 calorie per day diet. Includes all sugars, natural and added.

APPENDIX 2. The Mix Food Quality Index ™.

FOOD ITEMS	API	CSI	PDI	NIH	Mix Food Quality Index ™ Score
Spinach	4.00	5.07	1.30	1.97	**8.40**
Soybean	1.57	6.00	1.90	1.26	**8.21**
Wheat Germ	2.00	4.73	1.40	0.46	**7.67**
Broccoli	4.00	4.31	1.30	2.09	**7.52**
Flaxseed	1.10	5.59	1.31	0.82	**7.18**
Tomato	3.00	4.20	1.20	1.51	**6.89**
Salmon	1.73	4.22	2.00	1.22	**6.73**
Red Pepper	3.11	3.45	1.05	1.26	**6.35**
Almond	1.16	4.44	1.38	0.87	**6.11**
Carrot	3.09	4.07	0.80	2.09	**5.87**
Orange	2.11	4.07	0.63	1.00	**5.81**
Cabbage	2.44	4.06	1.30	2.10	**5.70**
Peanut	1.45	3.85	1.50	1.32	**5.48**
Onion	1.52	4.07	0.93	1.22	**5.30**
Corn	1.45	3.58	1.40	1.41	**5.02**
Chicken (no skin)	1.13	2.77	2.00	1.06	**4.84**
Sweet Potato	2.27	3.70	0.68	1.85	**4.80**
Egg	1.93	2.84	2.00	2.22	**4.55**
White Potato (with skin)	1.16	3.26	0.85	0.77	**4.50**
Chicken (with skin)	1.27	2.70	2.00	1.49	**4.48**
Grape	1.49	2.83	0.38	1.13	**3.57**
Apple (with skin)	1.54	2.61	0.23	1.08	**3.30**
Hamburger	1.20	2.19	2.00	2.35	**3.04**
Hot Dog	0.98	1.75	1.91	2.42	**2.22**
French Fries	0.51	3.45	0.32	2.07	**2.21**
Candy (M&M's)	0.34	2.56	0.23	2.67	**0.46**

APPENDIX 3. World Health Organization Recommendations For Diet and Nutrition*

Dietary Factor	Goal (% of total energy, unless otherwise stated)
Total Fat	15 - 30%
Saturated fatty acids	<10%
n-6 Polyunsaturated fatty acids (PUFAs)	5 - 8%
n-3 Polyunsaturated fatty acids (PUFAs)	1 - 2%
Trans fatty acids	<1%
Monounsaturated fatty acids (MUFAs)	by difference[1]
Total Carbohydrate	55 - 75%[2]
Free sugars[3]	<10%
Protein	10 - 15%[4]
Cholesterol	<300 mg per day
Sodium chloride (sodium)[5]	<5 g per day (<2 g per day)
Fruits and vegetables	>400 g per day
Total dietary fiber	10 - 13 grams per 1000 calories (20 - 26 g day)

1. This is calculated as: total fat -- (saturated fatty acids + polyunsaturated fatty acids + trans fatty acids).

2. The percentage of total energy available after taking into account that consumed as protein and fat, hence the wide range.

3. The term "free sugars" refers to all monosaccharides and disaccharides added to foods by the manufacturer, cook or consumer, plus sugars naturally present in honey, syrups and fruit juices.

4. The suggested range should be seen in the light of the Joint WHO/FAO/UNUExpert Consultation on Protein and Amino Acid Requirements in Human Nutrition, held in Geneva from 9 to 16 April 2002 (2).

5. Salt should be iodized appropriately (6). The need to adjust salt iodization, depending on observed sodium intake and surveillance of iodine status of the population, should be recognized.

* World Health Organization Technical Report Series. "Diet, Nutrition, and the Prevention of Chronic Diseases" Report of a Joint FAO/WHO Consultation. Geneva. 2003.p.66. Available online at:

http://whqlibdoc.who.int/trs/WHO_TRS_916.pdf.

Accessed November 19, 2008.

APPENDIX 4. Basic Recommendations from ACSM and AHA*

Guidelines for healthy adults under age 65

Do moderately intense cardio 30 minutes a day,

five days a week

Or

Do vigorously intense cardio 20 minutes a day, 3 days a week

And

Do eight to 10 strength-training exercises,

eight to 12 repetitions of each exercise twice a week

Moderate-intensity physical activity means working hard enough to raise your heart rate and break a sweat, yet still being able to carry on a conversation. It should be noted that to lose weight or maintain weight loss, 60 to 90 minutes of physical activity may be necessary. The 30-minute recommendation is for the average healthy adult to maintain health and reduce the risk for chronic disease.

*Physical Activity and Public Health Guidelines, American College of Sports Medicine and the American Heart Association, American College of Sports Medicine website, http://www.acsm.org//AM/Template.cfm?Section=Home_Page, Accessed November 21, 2008.

APPENDIX 5. Additional Resources.

BOOKS

- Bowman, B. and Russell, R. *Present Knowledge in Nutrition,* 9th edition, volumes I and II. Washington, D.C.: International Life Sciences Institute, 2006.

- Cooper, K. *Antioxidant Revolution.* Nashville: Thomas Nelson Publishers, 1993.

- Erasmus, U. *Fats that Heal; Fats that Kill.* Vancouver: Alive Books, 1993.

- Gruenwald, J., Brendler T., and Jaenicke C, eds. *PDR for Herbal Medicines,* 4th edition. Montvale, NJ: Thomson Healthcare, 2007.

- Hobbs, C. *Echinacea: The Immune Herb.* Santa Cruz: Botanica Press, 1996.

- Ody, P. The Complete Herbal. Milan: Dorling Kindersley, 1993.

- Pawlak, L. *A Perfect 10: Phyto "New-trients" against Cancers.* Emeryville, CA: Biomed General Corp., 1998.

- Tyler, V.E. *Herbs of Choice: The Therapeutic Use of Phytomedicinals.* Binghamton, NY: Pharmaceutical Products Press, 1994.

- Tyler, V.E. *The Honest Herbal: A Sensible Guide to the Use of Herbs and Related Remedies.* Binghamton, NY: Pharmaceutical Products Press, 1993.

WEB RESOURCES

- American Botanical Council.

  http://www.herbalgram.org

- American Dietetic Association.

  http://www.eatright.org

- American College of Sports Medicine.

  http://www.acsm.org

- American Heart Association.
  http://www.americanheart.org

- American Herbal Products Association.
  http://www.ahpa.org

- Institute of Medicine.
  http://www.iom.edu

- Linus Pauling Institute, Oregon State University.
  http://lpi.oregonstate.edu

- The National Academies.
  http://www.nas.edu

- USDA Nutrient Data Laboratory.
  http://www.nal.usda.gov/fnic/foodcomp/search

- World Health Organization.
  http://www.who.int/en

www.ingramcontent.com/pod-product-compliance
Lightning Source LLC
Chambersburg PA
CBHW031931190326
41519CB00007B/489